FEDERAL-STATE HEALTH POLICIES AND IMPACTS:

The Politics of Implementation

Christa Altenstetter
City University of New York
and Wissenschaftszentrum--Berlin

and

James Warner Bjorkman
University of Wisconsin-Madison

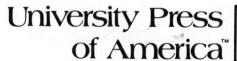

University Press
of America™

Copyright © 1978 by

University Press of America, Inc.™

4710 Auth Place, S.E., Washington, D.C. 20023

ISBN: 0-8191-0503-1

Library of Congress Catalog Card Number: 78-62173

PREFACE

From 1972 to 1976, an interdisciplinary research team at the Yale School of Medicine investigated the impact of federal initiatives on state health policy formation and service delivery patterns. The Yale Health Policy Project was funded by grant number 5-R01-HS-00900 from the Department of Health, Education and Welfare's National Center for Health Services Research and Development, a division of the Health Resources Administration within the U.S. Public Health Service. As the political scientists on our interdisciplinary project, we presented an initial draft of our policy findings at the 1977 annual meeting of the American Political Science Association. This book represents a substantially elaborated and refined final version of our study.

During the years past we have extensively utilized the files of the Health Policy Project, the support of whose staff is gratefully acknowledged. In particular we would like to thank our colleagues -- Milton Chen, Anne-Marie Foltz, Daniel Friedman and especially George Silver, who contributed the foreword -- for their persistent advice and tenacious arguments that tempered but did not blunt our conclusions. We, of course, remain responsible for the latter and for whatever sins of omission or commission lead to them.

We must also thank our many talented research assistants -- William Averyt, James Grisolia, Michael Halle, Barbara Novak, Eric Peterson, Kim Rosenfield, Elizabeth Stevens, Alan Stoga, and Natalie Tyler -- whose painstaking, time-consuming labors over the four years permitted us to collect sufficient historical information to trace the temporal dimension in American child-health policy. Likewise we are unusually endebted to a series of patient, persevering typists -- Beth Lorenzi and Barb Hall at Yale; and Marge Kritz and Becky Richards at Wisconsin -- who tolerated seemingly innumerable incarnations of our edited and re-edited prose. Certainly without the keen eye and sure touch of Ms. Richards, the current manuscript would still be a pile of disjointed notes and indecipherable jottings.

Those to whom we owe the greatest thanks, however, must go unnamed. In Connecticut and Vermont as well as in Boston and Washington, dozens of interviewees set aside hours of valuable time to explain their versions of what really happened during the implementation of a public policy. While reserving personal responsibility for the information and interpretations in this monograph, we wish to thank them collectively within the ethical limits set by the code of confidentiality.

CA & JWB

June, 1978

iv

FOREWORD

As the complexities of modern medical practice
generate more and more difficulties for attaining
such social goals as equity, quality care or cost
containment, more attention is being paid the role of
the federal government in achieving control over this
apparently unmanageable sector. It is clear that the
federal government itself cannot supervise or manage
such a vast and multivariate industry, with such
large numbers of variously trained workers in so many
different institutional settings, so the question
of decentralized controls and delegation of responsibility comes to the fore. The federal-state relationship thus lies at the heart of the matter.
However, as the current evidence plainly shows, our
federal-state system fails to produce a satisfactory
implementation of public policy goals. This short-
fall is, of course, not only true of the health
system but also of other systems that rely on that
federal-state relationship as well.

Because national involvement in the health
system -- or rather in the medical care system, since
we have hardly any investment in health as such in
this country -- is relatively recent, identifying
the causative factors that produce these deficiencies
in implementation may not be too difficult. The
wounds are still close to the surface. And if the
nature of the difficulties can be identified and the
causes spelled out, it is not unlikely that effective
measures can also be designed to correct them. In
that case, the medical care system may serve as a
guide to the reform and reconstruction of other
federal-state arrangements.

This book deals with a specific case study of
child health services, which depend heavily on
federal funding and state action. The evidence is
incontrovertible that except for the fact that the
federal exchequer supplied the funds, state actions

were dictated by state rather than federal policies. Furthermore, the national concern did not emerge in any of the policy arenas where one might have expected that control and supervision would be exercised: the Congress and the Executive Branch. In a word, federal-state actions were neither joint nor collaborative.

Since the purpose of the original legislation was to promote a national policy, the lack of effective impact of federal policy on a state's actions represents a significant failure of American legislative and social philosophy. Yet because the future well-being of the country and its citizens will depend heavily on successful federal-state action, and not only in the field of health and medical care, it is important to search the following implementation analysis for keys to how the situation might be modified. Recommending more supervision is naive, since the structure obviously obstructs this approach. But experiments with completely decentralized activity, perhaps even with local rather than federal funding, along with a strong, built-in legal protection in the hands of the local citizens, may produce a more powerful tool and a more useful method to ensure satisfactory services than to create another national program. Of course, lying in the way of achieving this objective today is a long history of federal preemption of local authority as well as the general weakness of state and local governments in carrying out public policies. Nevertheless, it is clear that federal funding without large scale supervisory actions (the latter very expensive and hardly feasible for a country of our size and population) will not accomplish national goals either.

In short, this important document underlines the failure of federal policy to have an impact on state policy in child health, a failure in the implementation of national policy which may only be redressed by a totally new view of and approach to local government.

George A. Silver, M.D.
Professor of Public Health
Yale School of Medicine
New Haven, Connecticut

May, 1978

TABLE OF CONTENTS

LIST OF TABLES

LIST OF TABLES (Continued)

LIST OF ACRONYMS

ACD   - Aid to Dependent Children

AFDC - Aid to Families with Dependent
        Children

AMA   - American Medical Association

CCS   - Crippled Children's Services

C&Y   - Children and Youth

D/HEW - Department of Health, Education
        and Welfare

EPSDT - Early and Periodic Screening,
        Diagnosis and Treatment

MCH   - Maternal and Child Health

M&I   - Maternal and Infant Care

OEO   - Office of Economic Opportunity

PHN   - Public Health Nurses

SRU   - Summer Round-Up

WCC   - Well Child Clinic/Conference

Chapter I

Federal-State Relations: Tensions and Opportunities for Implementation

Tensions and conflicts exist among partners in any federal polity. Problems in setting, financing and implementing policy priorities reemphasize the need to clarify relationships within the intergovernmental system as well as interdependencies among governmental *and* non-governmental organizations. The degree and quality of these linkages are vital areas of research not only on federalism and the component parts of the federal system but also on policy implementation and policy management in the national political system.

A recent concern among policy makers is building the capacity of state and local governments to manage federal problems. This concern about interdependencies within the federal polity derives from different streams of thought, perspectives and research activities. The research community and the policy actors, regardless of their different methodologies and levels of abstraction, share a common concern about policy analysis. And their concern centers around a desire to better understand the dynamics of the intergovernmental system as it affects the implementation of national objectives, to propose and test hypotheses about causal linkages in the implementation process, and to develop a reliable framework for predicting policy impacts in future programs based on assessments of alternative administrative strategies.

Less prompted by theory than by practice, a new appreciation of intergovernmental relations as an evolutionary process and a pragmatic art of governing a federally structured political system has emerged. Gaps often appear between the proclamation and the achievement of policy goals because governmental mechanisms are often wasteful, duplicative and archaic. Even so, domestic policies increasingly rely on the intergovernmental system for implementation and thus produce greater interdependencies among all public and private components of the national system.

In order to translate policy demands into tangible benefits through effective, efficient and equitable implementation, three requirements are necessary. First, economic resources must be available. Second, both governmental and non-governmental organizations are needed to supply the administrative framework. And third, skilled and experienced manpower must be on tap to carry out policy goals. Each set of resources has a different impact on the implementation of government policies.

Furthermore, the relative presence or absence of these resources has stimulated conflict within the intergovernmental system. Tensions occur if one partner has disproportionate economic resources, or more organizational resources at a particular point in time, or better manpower skills in the public and private sectors; and the ensuing conflicts have been important sources of governmental change throughout American history. As a modernizing nation the United States has repeatedly attempted to reconcile tensions over these three sets of variables. Consequently a growing network of inter-organizational and intra-organizational relations developed; the texture of interactions among organizational personnel changed; and public and private governance became increasingly complex. Although America is areally organized, the dynamic effects of economic resources, organizational mechanisms, and professional-bureaucratic relations have transcended territorial boundaries.

The increasing interdependence of territorially organized governmental arenas is reflected in an ever larger share of federal grants-in-aid funds in state budgets and a larger share of state grants-in-aid in local government budgets. Prior to revenue-sharing, the intergovernmental grant device had been *the* most important change agent in the system, and often restructured state and local program priorities and decision-making hierarchies (Walker, 1974). Even after the introduction of revenue-sharing, budget interdependencies remain basic realities of the American federal system -- although such interdependency does not always mesh with cherished political myths and rhetoric about the constitutional autonomy of governmental levels.

Federal outlays to private recipients also have blurred the lines between public and private economic sectors. According to one recent study, "Private enterprise in America collects roughly $30 billion a year in government subsidies and subsidy-like aid, much of it hidden or disguished. .... Contrary to the conventional wisdom that private business is free of federal handouts, the study showed that it collects aid in many forms: cash payments, tax breaks, bargain-basement loans, technical guidance, low-cost services, and grants routed through state and municipal middlemen" (Shaw, 1973: 48).

Historically, federal assistance to state and local governments and/or private recipients has not only steadily increased, but also changed its form. Types of intergovernmental fiscal transfers have changed, different patterns of politics over the competition for funds have evolved, different administrative arrangements have been worked out among intergovernmental actors, and different access points for interest group demands became available. Accordingly, scholars of American government have classified the history of federal-state-local relations into several phases, each characterized by a particular pattern of politics, by a predominant mode of intergovernmental transfers of funds, and by a different mix of actors involved (ACIF, 1974; Beer, 1973; Elazar *et al.*, 1972; Grodzins, 1966; Leach, 1970; Wright, 1974).

3

The most dramatic changes in the mode of financing governmental tasks occurred in the mid-'30s. At that time, the practice of conducting government business by financing activities mainly from resources raised by the respective level of government shifted to a financial mode in which combined tax resources raised by state and local governments were supplemented by federal grants-in-aid. The federal approach adopted in the '30s was one of providing categorical grants for specific purposes and earmarked for target population groups and areas. By the '60s categorical grants had been complemented with project and block grants. And by 1975, the intergovernmental fiscal system was based on three main pillars: revenue sharing, block grants, and categorical grants. However, while few policy areas are implemented through any one single method of financing, a salient feature of this tri-part approach is that categorical grants still account for about three-quarters of federal assistance to the states (ACIR, 1975:3).

The history of the United States has been one of expanding organizational resources and changing institutional relationships, and the period after World War II was particularly marked by intense institution-building for government services. Today, in addition to the federal government and the fifty state governments, there are 18,000 general purpose municipalities, 17,000 general purpose townships, more than 3,000 county governments, and 24,000 special purpose districts. In order to coordinate this plethora of governmental units at various levels, many new regional arrangements have been innovated. Much of the institution-building in the '60s to bridge the organizational interstices was federally initiated but with considerable local consequences. In some cases, regional arrangements started from scratch; in others, old institutions (public and/or private) were rejuvenated and given a different mandate; and in still others, some blend of new and old mechanisms can be discerned. In all cases, however, these public organizations are also involved in the business of formulating and implementing policies (ACIR, 1975).

4

Agencies at various levels of government, however, are not the only organizational resources available for implementing policies. Many non-profit and private agencies also perform public functions with public funds through government-by-contract. Since the '60s these, too, have increased considerably in number and significance for policy implementation.

In addition to economic and organizational resources, skilled and experienced manpower resources are vital for implementation. Constituency building and coalition formation within highly specialized public and private bureaucracies are well-known phenomena. In an intergovernmental and inter-organizational context, the use of the grants-in-aid device since the '30s has intensified the exchange of information among functional specialists in all areas of human activity. Similar training and skills have facilitated communication among the intergovernmental professional guilds and with their peers in private organization. Communications flow from functional specialists in the federal system to functional specialists in the states and localities, or vice versa; and communications across state and community boundaries have facilitated the permeation of the political system by the interests of diverse professional groups. Such patterns of communication clearly transcend any boundaries set up by bureaucratic and/or jurisdictional hierarchies.

In the following chapters, by investigating the fate of several federal-state child-health programs, we examine the interplay among these sets of economic, organizational and personnel resources within the American intergovernmental system. After the context and background of our comparative case-studies are introduced in Chapter II, three subsequent chapters discuss a series of policy impacts (direct, indirect, and interactive) and how over time the unfolding implementation process produced such results. The concluding chapter generalizes about how public policies, once enunciated, are likely to be refashioned when implemented through an intergovernmental system. In an era when burgeoning numbers of social problems appear on the public agenda and when federal interventions increasingly occur across a range of substantive policies, our findings should be both sobering and challenging.

Chapter II

American Child Health Policy:
Background and Methodology of a Case Study

Introduction:

Federal initiatives in health care have produced
increasingly visible and important intergovernmental
impacts. Annual federal health care investments have
tripled to over $30 billion during the past decade,
and health-related expenditures by governments at all
levels approach $60 billion each year. Public expen-
ditures now account for 40 percent of annual health-
care costs in the United States. Consequently,
changes have occurred in relationships between
federal and state governments as well as between the
public and private sectors, even as new interest
groups surface in areas long dominated by well-
established groups. And between such initiatives
and their impacts lies the ill-charted realm of
policy implementation.

At the same time, the cumulative intergovernmental impacts, whether shifts over influence or
access to public funds, have roots in prior policies
which encouraged private health care. Despite
dramatic inflations in sums and percentages, many
features of the nation's health system display more
continuity than change. This monograph explores
some of the political and administrative lessons
that can be learned from how states respond to
federal initiatives in health care.

There are many health policies in the US which could reveal the influence of federal initiatives on the several states, but most are fairly complex and of recent origin. Child-care itself, of course, is not a narrow social policy because children today comprise about 40 percent of the American population; indeed the health of America's children is rhetorically acknowledged as important for the nation's long-term well-being and safety (Bjorkman and Kinsey, 1973; Keniston, 1974; Silver, 1975; Steiner, 1976). But an examination of child health programs has several advantages. The impact of federal child-care programs on state health policy conveniently spans the range of policy studies (Froman, 1968) because the topic simultaneously deals with the health (substantive category) of children (target category) during the last forty years (time category), and how presumably good (value category) social welfare aims (ideological category) are affected by other governmental relations (institutional category). Several major studies of federal child health programs have been completed (Huron Institute, 1972; George Washington University, 1973; Kakalik *et al.*, 1973 and 1974; and Davis, 1975) which vary considerably in scope and methodology. Most use survey and interview methods to inventory programs, but none focus explicitly on political factors and processes.

American child health policy is expressed in a number of federal legislative enactments, the most comprehensive of which is the Social Security Act. Federal initiatives on behalf of maternal and child health began in 1923 with the Sheppard-Towner Act, but that experiment lapsed in 1929. The Social Security Act, passed in 1935 as part of the New Deal, included among its provisions a commitment to promote the health and well-being of mothers, infants, and disadvantaged children in rural and economically depressed areas. The categorical programs authorized were Maternity and Child Health (MCH) and Crippled Children's Services (CCS), which collectively comprised Title V of the Act. The MCH package included well-child conferences, dental hygiene education, pre-natal counseling, public health nursing, licensing and inspection; and the CCS package included case finding, diagnosis, and treatment of diseases leading to crippling conditions.

The Social Security Act has been repeatedly amended and expanded since 1935, most notably during the Great Society years of Lyndon Johnson's Administration. New projects for promoting maternal and child health in low-income areas were authorized such as Maternity and Infant Care (M&I) in 1963 and Children and Youth (C&Y) in 1965. Also in 1965, Title XIX was added which consolidated provisions from Titles I, IV, XIV, and XVI, and which sought to extend services to all needing financial help in meeting their medical obligations (Stevens and Stevens, 1974). The new Medicaid title established criteria of eligibility so that in addition to persons authorized to receive direct welfare payments (the indigent, all children under 21 who need but cannot afford medical care, and all AFDC families without fathers), those families who need help with excessive medical bills (the medically indigent) could also receive assistance. Furthermore, in 1968 a special amendment required the states to intensify efforts to screen and treat children with disabling conditions through early case-finding and periodic screening of children. The desultory impact of the Early and Periodic Screening, Diagnosis, and Treatment (EPSDT) amendments to Titles V and XIX is ably discussed in Foltz (1975) and in Foltz and Brown (1976). Although these recent additions to the Social Security Act provide by far the largest amount of federal funds going into the American states on behalf of children today, we are primarily interested in the long-term development and fate of the original programs. Longitudinal studies reveal broad patterns of impacts that the recent programs, although more detailed, cannot because of their brief operations.

Framework and Methodology:

In order to compare underlying methods of implementation and to assess changes in state laws and administrative organization, we concentrated on the major programs authorized by Title V. The impacts of these federally initiated child-care programs were traced through case studies of Connecticut and Vermont. Case studies, of course, provide too limited an empirical base for generalizing about federal impacts on the American states, but single cases are very useful in refining hunches into

9

hypotheses. And such hypotheses can later be examined in other contexts with comparative data.

Our initial objective had been to examine the impact of federal child health policy on state activities during the 1960s. But for Title V programs, the conflicts and solutions during the formative years following the passage of the Social Security Act had had an enduring effect on program intentions and operations. For example, Congress had legislated some minimum requirements before a state could receive funds through federal programs. In order to meet these federal requirements, states adjusted their legislative and executive arrangements in the 1930s, adjustments which still provide the bases for cooperative arrangements with the federal government.

In addition, many program procedures and standards of health care were institutionalized in the 1930s. During the New Deal, government reformers were interested in professionalizing public service, so the child-health programs were staffed with professionals. Today, many participants on professional advisory and supervisory committees derive their legitimacy from agreements obtained in the 1930s. Even in the new child-care programs added in the 1960s, well-established interest groups had automatic access to decision-making dating from agreements in previous decades while other groups were automatically overlooked or excluded. The formulation and supervision of health policy are clear examples of non-decision-making (Bachrach and Baratz, 1963), the impact of which is as real and consequential as acts of commission.

In other areas, the states had ample discretionary power to define eligibility, services to be rendered, outreach efforts, referral policies, and the extent of private cooperation. In these areas, pre-existing practices and philosophies and predominant state attributes made an imprint on program operations. As the analysis will show, health officials in Vermont and Connecticut responded quite differently to the challenge of formulating 'progressive' or 'conservative' health policies for the respective target population. But both dovetailed their programs into the prevailing private health care system.

Federal child health policy, like other social policies, is often unclear and subject to reinterpretation. Such ambiguity is partly due to imprecise Congressional objectives, but it derives partly from the process by which legislative intent is clarified -- or even specified -- by federal administrators. Over the years of Title V operations, for example, the responsible federal agency supplemented and elaborated its program mandate in ways not always congruent with original Congressional aspirations. Through regulations, administrators of the Children's Bureau specified fiscal and technical procedures; defined goals as if a national consensus existed which not even Congress was able to articulate; exceeded Congressional intentions by enlarging goals; reflected the public 'mood' as when the World Health Organization's 1949 Charter definition of health was adopted verbatim in 1949; and promoted goals not directly related to health such as the administrative reform movement of the 1930s. In all cases, however, the states could always count on the Bureau administering an ambiguous, flexible policy that allowed much state-level variation.

Comparative analysis of health care programs authorized by a single piece of legislation and operating under similar federal conditions has several advantages. Interstate comparison permits support, modification or rejection of findings drawn from a single case study. The case experience of Vermont serves as a critical test of our tentative conclusions about federal impact in Connecticut (Altenstetter and Bjorkman, 1974). It also allows the identification of more causal factors and an explanation of differential performances under MCH and CCS in both states.

Although the impacts of Title V's MCH and CCS programs were traced historically in both states from 1935 to 1975, no single approach could provide an adequate conceptual framework to encompass all our comparative studies. The research topics, both theoretically and empirically, spanned time, territory, administrative forms, political subdivisions, group politics, and fiscal transfers. The field of policy analysis is still fragmented into many competing methodologies and the field of intergovernmental relations is itself amorphous. We therefore surveyed the literature on policy science

11

and program evaluation, on state and local politics, on federalism and redistributive financing, on bureaucracy and public administration. Other broad areas examined were economic decision-making, interest group activities and public health.

These analytic topics, in turn, suggested diverse roles, conflicts, solutions, linkages, and relationships which may exist among public and private actors and institutions. We would be the last to argue that all these foci can be amalgamated into or subsumed under a single analytic framework, because politics and policy remain too rich and varied for gross simplification. But some attempts at configurational analysis are *sine qua non* for any adequate policy study, and from these initial investigations four broad interactive areas of inquiry emerged for consideration. Governmental relations, program delivery systems, expenditure patterns, and private interests have served as vantage points for exploring, understanding, and explaining the policy implementation process illustrated by the child health programs.

The downward flow of federal initiatives were first examined as expressed in law, appropriations, and administrative regulations. These intergovernmental relations were supplemented by intragovernmental relations among units of government at each level (nation, region, state, district, locality), and soon patterns of reciprocal impact and feedback began to appear. Included in our study of the program delivery system were administrative control over state health services; the decentralized units which deliver direct services; and the program personnel who run the programs or are reimbursed after providing health care. Since the Social Security Act required states to match federal monies under varying formulas, expenditure patterns necessarily focussed attention on the origin of funds, and on estimates about income transfers. In addition, private interests permeate the governmental process and appear particularly significant for health policy implementation at the state level.

Because there are several kinds of impact, analyses of intergovernmental policy face difficulties of operational measurement. Other than being identified in the broadest terms, various political, administrative, and fiscal impacts are difficult to specify. And since relationships in a federal system are rarely unidirectional, reciprocity remains a problem. Furthermore, historical experiences have a cumulative effect on the achievement of policy goals, a cumulative experience which needs to be evaluated in order to understand the present.

For convenience in discussion, federal-state impacts can be classified as direct, indirect, and interactive. Direct impacts compare service outputs of federal child health programs with stated Congressional intentions. This comparison of goals and achievements most closely approximates the conventional understanding of an evaluative methodology for policy analysis. The underlying aim is to assess program efficiency by discovering whether explicit goals were achieved and, if so, at what cost per unit.

For Title V the legislative goals were operationalized as federal share of state program budgets; number of children served; rural placement of clinics; and the stimulation of employment opportunities. Of course, the amount of money spent on government programs is an incomplete measure of policy outcomes. The conceptualization of state policy in terms of the amount of dollars allocated to a particular issue area, while distinctly conducive to empirical measurement, has come under increasing criticism. As Schaefer and Rakoff (1970: 61) observe, the model "suffers from its oversimplification of complex phenomena, its tendency to substitute ease of measurement for conceptual rigor, and the fact that it has been (and perhaps can only be) applied to the analysis of expenditure policy."

Since Congress is justifiably concerned with how federal dollars are used, this policy-dollars measure is even more questionable in the field of intergovernmental relations. Direct measures of services specified in federal law were therefore included, but with the understanding that even these are not fully adequate. Congressional intentions vary widely, and federal appropriations may, for example, finance tangible goods and services for a clearly defined target population. On the other hand, they may underwrite programs which are intended to enhance the

13

ability of a state to achieve a further goal. Even more perplexingly, although they may be intended to improve the health of children, federal monies may also be used to balance centripetal and centrifugal forces in American federalism. The field of inter-governmental relations explicitly recognizes that although the levels of American government interpene-trate in 'marbled fashion', federal, state, and local governments emphasize different goals, have different value orientations and traditions, and involve dif-ferent mixes of actors (Grodzins, 1966; Elazar, 1972; Ostrom, 1973). Therefore, there are wide ranges of motives for and receptivity to federal policy priori-ties.

Beyond the provision of direct services, federal initiatives also influence a state's administrative capabilities. An important, although often unstated, distinction in the social policy field is between maintenance and opportunity policies (Morehouse, 1972: 9-12). Maintenance policies seek to provide a target population with goods and services which are in themselves immediately beneficial; their outcomes are terminal in that they are consumed by the benefi-ciaries. On the other hand, opportunity policies seek to enhance the ability of a target group (or, more usually, an institution or agency) to provide goods or services to others; these outcomes are instrumental because they lead to future payoffs. Whereas maintenance policies are oriented toward tangible results, opportunity policies are oriented toward improving process for they latter intend to expand administrative capabilities. Such indirect impact is instrumental for it changes the organiza-tional structure in which child health programs operate.

The problem with opportunity policies, however, is that the outcomes of such changes are not always predictable, or even anticipated. As one example, federal policy on the merit system led to increased influence of health professionals in the Title V programs. There was, however, no clear understanding of how and to whom these new powerholders could be held accountable. Ultimately informal peer group relationships among medical professionals became more important than public accountability to consumers of health care.

14

Indirect impacts are even more difficult to measure and assess than direct impacts. Although any 'policy' includes both initial goal and supplementary practices (Lasswell and Kaplan, 1950: 71), these tend to change over time. Public policies in particular are continuously reinterpreted and modified, amplified and/or restricted at successive levels of government. New rules for actions may supercede or coexist with old behavioral parameters. New goals may emerge from a change in value perspectives. In addition, changes in public policy at one level of government influence performance at other levels, whether federal, state or local. Hence neither formal rules nor informal procedures remain static.

Formalized rules for action include federal laws, federal executive regulations, state laws, state administrative regulations, state health plans and other directive guidelines. These rules shape the implementation process in federal child health policies by providing a framework for the health care delivery system; they also influence interest group behavior. In addition to formal rules, policy content is molded by administrative practice. An apparently explicit policy may become progressively more ambiguous as successive implementation decisions contradict one another. In general, the more rule-makers there are, the higher the potential for redefining and changing policy. This obvious, but often neglected, point is particularly significant for studying the formulation and implementation of public policies in a federal system.

Finally, in addition to direct service impacts and indirect organizational impacts, federal policy can shape and reshape the political system itself. Depending on one's vantage point, such impacts are both reciprocal and reflexive since a federal system has, almost by definition, continual interaction among levels of government. Such interactions are often ignored or assumed to be unidirectional. Yet in actual practice, state receptivity and local predispositions toward federal initiatives are potential determinants of change in federal policy. The political dynamics of intergovernmental relations may complicate the analysis of policy impacts, but such dynamics also reveal how a particular state can mold the contents of federal policies.

15

A word of caution is in order, however, whether impacts are regarded as direct, indirect, or inter-active. Ambiguous goals necessarily hamper efforts to evaluate any impacts of social policies, and the Title V programs are no exception to this rule. Programs with broad aims have elusive results which make intended effects hard to locate and measure. Also, considering the distinction between latent and manifest function, even programs with specific inten-tions can produce unexpected consequences. Most policy analyses presume clarity of purpose, a pre-sumption of dubious value in social policy studies. As a prominent US Senator's legislative aide put it: "Anything you can do to show that the policy process is less orderly and regular than we think is a contribution in the direction of truth."

Connecticut and Vermont: A Comparative Profile

Before discussing the impacts of federal child health policy in Connecticut and Vermont, the two states should be briefly compared. The environmental context provides a background against which the similarities and differences of program performance must be interpreted. While Connecticut and Vermont vary in society, economy and politics, they share a long, common tradition of local town government. Indeed, Vermont's earliest settlers and leaders came primarily from Connecticut's Litchfield County, and for a brief time they called their settlement New Connecticut. In contrast with intraregional varia-tions elsewhere in the United States, both states have also shared in the historical development of New England, the oldest region of the nation (Lockard, 1956; Sharkansky, 1970). As but one consequence, Vermont and Connecticut are both served by the same regional office of the US Department of Health, Education, and Welfare. Federal initiatives and responses are therefore channeled through the staff conduits of the New England Regional Office located in Boston.

But the two states also differ sharply, and not only because Connecticut has a sevenfold larger population. Connecticut and Vermont are, respec-tively, wealthly and impoverished; urban and rural; industrialized and agricultural; densely and sparsely populated. In addition, Vermont has long been a Republican stronghold while Connecticut reveals

16

reveal considerable partisan competitiveness. Connecticut's political parties are strong whereas Vermont's are loosely articulated and disorganized. And compared to the weak office of Governor in Vermont, the formal powers of Connecticut's Governor are relatively strong (Citizens Conference on State Legislatures, 1971).

In fiscal policies, other dimensions distinguish the two states. Vermont spends more in general per capita expenditures, yet ranks much lower on a welfare-education index. Connecticut relies on raising state revenues to finance highly professional staffs which Vermont does not. And Connecticut's fluid resources are subject to greater directive control by the state legislature and executive officials.

Table I: Comparative Characteristics

	Connecticut	Vermont
1970 Physicians/1000 population	1.91	1.87
1970 Hospital beds/1000 population	3.34	4.51
Per Capita Medicaid Expenditures		
1968	$19.66	$19.86
1970	$27.32	$27.95
1972	$34.67	$37.93
Title V Benefit/Cost Ratio		
1966 Total	.70	1.69
Federal	.61	3.01
State	.81	.94
1969 Total	.69	2.04
Federal	.67	4.32
State	.72	1.06

Source: Health Policy Project Files; and Cooper and Worthington, 1975: 24-26.

Nonetheless, the two states are remarkably similar in health resources. Despite demographic and financial disparities, Table I illustrates their 1970 parity in physician and hospital-bed ratios. Medicaid expenditure per capita was almost identical although Vermont obtained a considerably better benefit/cost ratio in its Title V programs. At least in recent years, the existing health programs work to better advantage in Vermont.

Chapter III

Policy Implementation: Direct Impacts

Finances

A major, or at least convenient, indicator of
federal impact on state level child health programs
is the proportion of a program's budget financed by
federal expenditures. Fiscal data are intuitively
simple measures of policy commitments and presumably
are easy to locate in a record-keeping society.
Surprisingly, however, comparative fiscal information on such well-established child health programs
as MCH and CCS has been difficult to find and to
validate (see Appendix A, Tables 1-6 for basic data,
sources, and explanatory notes).

Of the federal funds flowing into the two
states, aggregate health money never exceeds ten
percent of all annual federal grants to state and
local governments. At the same time, both

Table II: Comparative Fiscal Shares (by percent)

	US Health Grants / Total Federal Grants (all states)	Federal Health Aid / Health Expenditures (Connecticut only)	Federal Health Aid / Health Expenditures (Vermont only)
1940	3	5	45
1950	6	4	21
1960	3	6	43
1970	4	15	19

Source: Altenstetter, 1971: 62-64; and Bjorkman, 1975b.

19

Connecticut and Vermont obtain significant portions
of their fiscal resources for health programs from
Washington. And when funds for Medicare and
Medicaid are considered, the federal government
contributes almost half of each state's health-
related expenditures.

Since 1938 the magnitude of the annual federal
grants to both Title V programs in Connecticut has
increased more than fifteen-fold in current dollars.
As Table III demonstrates, even when inflation has
been controlled by calculating constant dollars, the
federal largesse has increased five times. Despite
some erratic jumps,the federal grants to Connecticut's MCH and CCS programs have steadily increased
by modest increments. Federal grants to Vermont
have also increased steadily and incrementally
during the past four decades but at a somewhat
slower rate. In current dollars Vermont's MCH
grants grew only six-fold and consequently, when

Table III: Federal Grants to Title V Programs

	MCH			
Year	Current $		Constant $	
	CT	VT	CT	VT
1937	41,223	23,313	92,636	52,984
1940	65,332	57,774	148,797	131,304
1945	64,800	51,812	108,543	86,353
1950	97,434	72,895	121,489	91,119
1955	130,314	71,102	143,360	78,134
1960	259,346	109,734	251,061	106,538
1965	445,223	137,635	401,608	123,995
1970	690,127	136,000	510,298	100,740
	CCS			
1937		12,217		27,766
1940	31,671	17,298	72,144	39,314
1945	79,345	15,916	132,906	26,527
1950	134,837	65,624	168,126	82,030
1955	191,172	64,037	210,310	70,370
1960	221,340	92,794	214,269	90,091
1965	353,990	172,121	319,197	155,064
1970	512,038		378,770	

Source: Appendix A.

20

inflationary effects are controlled, these federal grants to Vermont only doubled. The CCS grants, on the other hand, increased fourteen-fold in current dollars. The comparatively faster growth of Connecticut's federal grants is partly due to its more rapid demographic expansion because of urbanization and partly an artifact of Vermont's more extensive efforts at child care before the Social Security Act. Ironically, although the poorer state, Vermont had more infrastructure in place to accept and utilize the Title V programs in their initial phases.

Among other aims, New Deal social legislation sought to encourage American state governments to raise additional revenues for child health services. Since the interwar economic depression, American politics has reflected a belief that the federal government exists in order to provide seed money, redistribute wealth, and create initiatives to which the constituent states will then respond in order to attain self-sufficiency (Grodzins, 1960: 269; Derthick, 1970: 7). Table IV indicates that the record of Title V programs in stimulating state responses, however, has been ambiguous. Over the decades, the federal government has paid for an erratic share of the costs under the MCH and CCS programs, and even this annual federal share is deceptive. Soon after the programs began, the states learned that special new state appropriations were not needed in order to obtain federal matching funds. Rather, a state was permitted to aggregate its state and local expenditures on health affairs and to present their cumulative sum as its matching money (Friedman, 1974: 20). Consequently, although these formula grants were technically categorical programs, they were also a prototype of health revenue-sharing.

At the same time, the federal formula grants undoubtedly stimulated state activities and supplied financial resources for programming child health services. Connecticut, for example, did initiate a state program in 1937 in order to screen and treat crippled children -- although some efforts in the private sector such as Newington Hospital already existed. And Vermont, in conjunction with other federal grants for public health nursing, re-established a specialized division for maternal and child health within its Health Department.

21

Table IV: Federal Share of Title V Program Costs
(percentage of total expenditures)

| | MCH | | CCS | |
	Connecticut	Vermont	Connecticut	Vermont
1940	69*	76	40*	47
1945	54*	73	60*	51
1950	46*	39	66*	87
1955	61*	32	66*	55
1963	50	34*	50	74
1969	56	27*	44	71*

*Grant money rather than audited expenditure; grants inflate
percentages because, giving the state the benefit of the
doubt, complete disbursement of the federal allotment is
assumed.

Source: Appendix A.

It is not clear, however, that the formula-grant
device increased the state's willingness, much less
its ability, to raise additional resources for
maternal and child health programs. Stoga (1975: 39)
concludes that "although historically Connecticut
state expenditures are stimulated by federal grants-
in-aid, expenditures for health from state sources
are unaffected by federal dollars." One interpretation is that federal involvement in health policy
through formula grants has encouraged, or at least
allowed, states to contravene federal regulations
with apparent inpunity. Despite the annual rigama-
role of requiring regional office approval of state
health plans, federal criteria for obtaining state
matching funds have not been enforced. Indeed, the
annual budgets for individual Title V programs are
instead repeatedly juggled through supplemental
budgets, and the decisions about matching funds are
entirely departmental rather than part of the overall
state budgetary process.

Health Status

The explicit goal of Title V is to improve child
health (U.S. Stat. 74th Congress, 1935-36, Vol. 49,
Part I, *Public Laws*). Consequently, changes in the

health status of children should reveal the policy's effects over time. Health specialists advised that one indicator of federal impact might be changed in the infant mortality rate. But our first case-study found "no unambiguous link between federal initiative and child health status in Connecticut" despite controls between areas with and without M&I projects. Chen et al,(1975: 71-89) also comment that health-status indicators are not secure bases for policy planning. Eventually our comparison of direct service impacts included only the relative number of children served and the urban-rural locations of program clinics.

Analyses of federal guidelines for Title V program operations reveal that the federal government increasingly pursued 'opportunity' rather than 'maintenance' policies (Altenstetter, 1973; and Friedman, 1974). The Children's Bureau, which until its abolition in 1969 had responsibility for the MCH and CCS programs, increasingly sought to develop state-level administrative capabilities rather than to provide direct services. As a result, federal resources served to expand health departments, legitimize interest group participation in policy-making, and reinforce the contemporary pattern of private health care. Federal resources did not directly pay for medical care. Whether Congress intended to pursue these goals is obscure, although probable, because Congressional law-making is characterized by hidden agendas and logrolling rather than explicit policy designations (Bailey, 1950; Hinckley, 1971; Lowi, 1972; Redman, 1973).

In any case, the language of the law did express a direct goal of improved health care for mothers and children, however such health care may have been defined. The law explicitly mandated the delivery of MCH and CCS services in rural and economically depressed areas. So in the simple terms, how many children were served and where?

Services Delivery - Number of Children

In the 1930s, Connecticut already had a state-financed package of MCH programs underway. Although one of the few states not participating in the federal Sheppard Towner Act that operated between 1923 and 1929, Connecticut's Bureau of Maternal and

Child Hygiene had developed diverse program components. While the State Health Department did not provide pre- or post-natal clinics, direct family planning services, school health examinations, or dental and hearing examinations, its most important programs for direct child health services were the Well-Child Conferences (WCCs) and, until 1946, the Summer Round Ups (SRUs) of pre-school children.

When Congress passed the 1935 Social Security legislation, a modest child and maternal health program was also underway in Vermont. Vermont had participated in the Shephard-Towner Act and received its first federal grants in 1926, but no matching funds were voted by the legislature. Thus, the Division of Maternal and Infant Hygiene (created from the Division of Child Welfare) was limited to an annual operating budget of $5,000 granted by the federal government. Lacking funds for an extensive program, the Division established a demonstration district for field work in several towns in the St. Johnsbury area. A field nurse was employed who held mothers' classes, children's health conferences, and public clinics; she also made home visits. This demonstration program was subsequently extended although it continued to operate entirely on the annual Sheppard-Towner grant. When the federal authorization expired in 1929, the Vermont Assembly allocated an equivalent amount to maintain the program (Bjorkman, 1975b).

In 1933, participation in the federally sponsored public works program enabled Vermont to establish a Public Health Nursing Section (PHN). PHN has remained primarily responsible for MCH services in Vermont since the Title V program began. In 1935, Vermont prepared to receive federal funds which were expected to have a decisive effect in stimulating and expanding child health services. The MCH program provided the funds and the Public Health Nursing Section delivered the services.

The annual number of children treated in each state are compared in Table V with the respective child populations below five years of age in Connecticut and Vermont. Of course, these programs could not be expected to reach all children because private medical practice provided and continues to provide screening services for much of the population. However, we might expect a substantial

24

Table V: Children Examined by Well Child Conferences

Year	Target Category Aged 0-5 Years		Percentage Served by WCCs[*]	
	Connecticut	Vermont	Connecticut	Vermont
1925	146,277		3.1	
1930	132,289		3.7	
1935	110,573		5.8	
1940	112,708		8.5	
1945	164,643		2.7	
1950	201,093	41,941	2.5	12.0
1955	231,035	43,100[**]	2.2	12.0
1960	269,381	43,873	1.3	11.0
1965	270,499	41,766	0.9	10.0
1970	243,652	39,658	1.0	7.0

[*] Until 1945, children screened at the pre-school Summer Round Ups are combined with the WCC figures.

[**] Actual year is 1956.

Sources: *Connecticut State Department of Health Annual Report,* respective years 1923 through 1946; *Annual Administrative Report to the Governor,* respective years 1947 through 1972; "MCH Health Services Provided or Paid for by State or Local Official Public Health Agencies," respective years from 1946 through 1970; and Foltz and Sacks, 1974.

proportion of each state's child population to be examined. Well Child Clinics represent state attempts to establish widespread facilities for periodically inspecting, weighing, and immunizing children under five and for detecting and diagnosing their defects and illnesses.

Until 1964, Connecticut's child population under five steadily increased; it then began to decline. The percentage of children examined at WCCs increased erratically from 1923 to the Second World War, at which time, the federal government's Emergency and Infant Care Program (1943-49) came into effect. After this emergency program ended, the percentage of children seen at WCCs steadily decreased until by the late 1960s, less than one percent of Connecticut's children under five were examined by state-sponsored clinics.

In Vermont, proportionally more children were screened by MCH programs than in Connecticut, but even Vermont's performance record has deteriorated. Child population trends in Vermont have closely paralleled national patterns for its total number of children under five steadily increased until the mid-1960s and then began to decline marginally. But while twelve percent of Vermont's children aged 0-5 years were served at MCH clinics in 1950, the percertage had almost halved two decades later. By 1973, only six percent of children under five years of age were served by WCC's. This relative decline in WCC activities parallels a relative decline in Vermont's MCH program as a whole. Indeed, as Table VI suggests, the distribution of MCH efforts among WCCs, nursing services, and school health has remained almost identical over the past forty years. In all cases, WCCs in Vermont received low priority in program operations. As an eighteen year average during 1956-1973, 16 percent of children receiving MCH services received them through WCCs whereas 27 percent received nursing services and 54 percent school health services.

Table VI: Vermont Children Served by Various MCH Programs (by percent; percentages in parentheses represent distribution of services within only the MCH package)

Year	Children Under 21	Total Served by MCH Programs	Percentage Served by: All MCH Programs
1956	151,620	33,943	22 (100)
1960	159,236	33,506	21 (100)
1966	173,950	31,685	18 (100)
1970	183,760	22,977	12 (100)

26

Table VI: Continued

Year	WCC's	School Health Services [*]	Nursing Services	All Other MCH Services [**]
1956	4.6 (21)	11.7 (52)	5.6 (25)	0.4 (2)
1960	2.9 (14)	11.8 (56)	5.8 (27)	0.4 (3)
1966	3.2 (18)	10.0 (56)	4.6 (25)	0.2 (1)
1970	1.5 (12)	7.4 (59)	3.1 (25)	0.5 (4)

[*] School health services include physical examinations by physicians, visual and audial screening, dental screening, health inspections, TB examinations, and smallpox vaccinations.

[**] Other programs include dental treatment, general pediatric clinics, special clinics, mental retardation, child development, nursing, and maternity.

Source: Foltz and Sacks, 1974

Public programs provide access to health services for children whose health care needs cannot be satisfied in the private market. And at least one aim of Title V has been to stimulate state activities in the child health care delivery system through federal-state programs. Yet neither Connecticut nor Vermont has had an auspicious performance record in child health services. Although federal funds to MCH programs have been increasing, even after controlling for inflation each state's MCH program has served steadily declining percentages of children. Certainly proportionally more Vermont Children have received health services, and Vermont has engaged in a larger variety of ancillary MCH health services than Connecticut. In these respects, Title V's MCH program has had a more marked effect in Vermont. But financial disbursements, at least as measured here, do not produce better service records; indeed, increasing disbursements for MCH might be associated with diminished services.

If the payoffs over time of Title V's Maternal and Child Health program have been questionable, what has been the performance record of Title V's other major provision? According to average rates of prevalence reported in various medical studies, about seven percent of American children have some crippling defect (Wholey and Silver, 1966: 11-10; and Wallace, 1962: 269). If this medical estimate is applied to each state's child population, an unimpressive and ambivalent performance record for CCS services emerges although the federal initiatives stimulated Connecticut to start a state program for crippled children in 1937 and helped Vermont expand its efforts for the handicapped.

Table VII estimates the number of children with handicapping conditions at seven percent of all children under 21 any given year, and it calculates

Table VII: Approximate Performance Record of CCS in Connecticut and Vermont

Year	Population Under 21		Estimates of Handicapped Children	
	CT	VT	CT	VT
1940	371,065	131,194	25,957	9,184
1950	624,901	140,195	43,743	9,914
1960	943,773	159,236	66,064	11,146
1970	1,163,806	183,760	81,466	12,863

Year	Children Served by CCS		Percentage of Handicapped Served by CCS	
	CT	VT	CT	VT
1940	985		3.8	
1950	3,521	1,549	8.0	15.8
1960	3,642	2,553	5.5	22.9
1970	3,220	2,803	3.9	21.8

Source: Appendix A, Tables 2 and 4

the CCS performance record against this annual base-line. After three years of Title V operations, 3.8 percent of all Connecticut children assumed to be suffering from a defect were served by its CCS program. The highest percentage ever reached was attained in 1950 when a total of 3,521 children received care, yet 92 percent of the presumed target population's needs remained unmet. Since 1950, the percentage of children suffering from a crippling condition who have received care from the federal-state CCS program has steadily declined.

Vermont, on the other hand, produced a compara-tively higher performance record for its CCS program, a record which improved over time. Even the lowest percentage of Vermont children served was double the corresponding Connecticut figure. Despite general inflation over the last 20 years, Vermont has evidently been able to do more for its handicapped children than Connecticut.

Ironically, Vermont's accomplishments under this federal-state program were not without costs. Unlike Connecticut, when the Title V programs began opera-tions Vermont already had a program for children and adults afflicted by infantile paralysis. During the 1910s several severe poliomyelitus epidemics occured in Vermont, and in 1914 the state laboratory of hygiene began a pilot project to study the disease and to help rehabilitate its victims. Initially supported by anonymous donations,* the Infantile Paralysis Program eventually received state funds and became a major division of the State Health Department (Aycock, 1924: 307-311). Federal initia-tives under CCS proved to be a mixed blessing for

---

*The originator and major patron of the poliomyelitus research project was reputedly Emily Proctor, a spinster member of the Proctor family which owned Vermont's largest marble quarries and dominated its political machine (Yale Health Policy Project files, 21 August 1974, interview with the retired Program Director of the Vermont Association for the Crippled, Inc.).

this research and rehabilitation program. On the one
hand, increased financial resources allowed Vermont's
Poliomyelitus Division to increase its staff and
thereby process more children; on the other, Vermont
had to restrict the delivery of health services under
CCS to children because of the federal mandate. As
the Vermont State Board of Health lamented in 1937:
"This work has been circumscribed because of the
restrictions placed on Federal money for treatment
only of patients under 21 years of age" *(Thirty-first
Report of the State Board of Health,* 1936-1937, p. 7).

Service Delivery: Service Locations

Adequate placement of screening and treatment
clinics for Title V programs was another major goal
in the 1935 Social Security Act. Federal legislation
sought to improve maternal and child health services
in rural areas and other economically depressed
regions. Determining whether an area is or is not
rural, however, becomes surprisingly problematic
because the official operational definition has
changed with each decennial census. In order to
simplify comparisons over the decades in Table VIII,
towns with a density of less than one person per acre
in 1960 were classified as rural. Because of their
long-standing political importance, towns in New
England states are appropriate units for comparing
service-delivery achievements. Until 1965, representation in the lower house of the Connecticut and
Vermont General Assemblies was based on towns rather
than population (Ogle, 1970; Nuquist and Nuquist,
1966).

Table VIII: Rural Towns Served by MCH Well-Child
Conferences (by percent)

	Connecticut	Vermont
1940	68	30
1959	36	--
1960	--	75
1968	--	92
1971	36	--
1974	--	65
	(N=129)	(N-252)

Source: Appendix B, Table 1 and 2

30

The early years of the Connecticut MCH program did stress the provision of services in the rural sector, and the respective proportions of urban and rural towns equipped with WCC clinics demonstrate's certain congruence with federal intentions. The federal objective of providing special attention and remedial care to the rural sector was met. The number of Connecticut towns covered by WCCs had declined since the 1940s, but expanded in Vermont. Likewise the proportion of rural towns covered has diminished in Connecticut but increased in Vermont. Trend lines in the two states have clearly diverged over time,* and quite unfavorably to the wealthier state.

While the Well-Child Conferences were a welcome example of community resource mobilization in the 1930s, they fell far short of satisfying Connecticut's needs for a comprehensive preventive program of child health services. The 1963 and 1965 additions of special projects under Title V were attempts to alleviate this need in certain selected localities, and the screening and treatment program appended to Titles V and XIX in 1967 was another serious attempt to provide comprehensive health coverage for certain groups of needy children. But these programs have either been extremely localized, like M&I and C&Y, or like EPSDT they have been very slow in getting underway (Foltz, 1975). In no case can we demonstrate that the health status of Connecticut's children has been unequivocally improved because of a federal program.

Vermont's WCC clinics were adapted to the rural nature of the state from the beginning of Title V operations. Resident children from rural areas were the prime target group to receive MCH services. Vermont's definite interest in discovering whether rural children received services is evident because the state agency collected its WCC data by town of residence and not by location of WCCs. The concern for outreach is commendable, and the rural coverage in Vermont met federal intentions. One explanation is the standing division of labor in Vermont between the

---

*

Other Connecticut towns may have unilaterally sponsored some sort of well-child conference, but data on such local clinics are incomplete.

31

public health nurses, who still provide most MCH services in the rural areas, and the private visiting nurse associations (today also called home health agencies) who serve the urban areas.

The federal government also expected the new CCS program to find and treat crippled children in rural areas. As a direct result of federal initiatives, both states set up clinics for screening, diagnosis and care. Connecticut established several permanent hospital-based clinics and other temporary clinics for more specialized screening as needed; in all, a total of 60 different clinics have participated at one time or another in Connecticut's CCS program. One private hospital, the Newington Home for Crippled Children, had already specialized in treating the state's physically handicapped children, and from 1938 through 1943 it hosted a CCS clinic. Four additional hospital-based clinics opened in Connecticut in 1938, of which two were in rural towns and two in urban ones. As Table IX shows, three of these original five clinics actually served urban counties, but after 1943 the balance shifted so that the rural counties had four of the state's seven permanent CCS clinics.

Table IX: CCS Clinic Placements (Part One)

LOCATION OF CRIPPLED CHILDREN'S SERVICES IN CONNECTICUT

Opened	Town	County Service Area	Urban/Rural
Pre-1934	*Newington	Hartford	Urban
1936-1940	*Willimantic	Windham	Rural
	*Norwich	New London	Rural
	*Danbury	Fairfield	Urban
	*Stamford	Fairfield	Urban
Post-1940	*Putnam	Windham	Rural
	*Torrington	Litchfield	Rural

*Hospital-based clinics

Source: *Biennial Reports of the Connecticut and Vermont State Health Departments*, 1934-1974; *Connecticut State Register and Manual*, 1940 and Levenson, 1966; *Vermont Yearbooks*, 1935-1975; and interview files, Yale Health Policy Project.

Table IX: CCS Clinic Placements (Part Two)

LOCATION OF CRIPPLED CHILDREN'S SERVICES IN VERMONT

Opened	Town	County Service Area	Urban/Rural
Pre-	Barre	Washington	Rural
1934	Barton	Orleans	Rural
	*Burlington	Chittendon	Rural
	Montpellier	Washington	Rural
	Newport	Orleans	Rural
	Proctor	Rutland	Rural
	Rutland	Rutland	Rural
	St. Alban's	Franklin	Rural
	St. Johnsbury	Caledonia	Rural
	Windsor	Windsor	Rural
1936-	Bennington	Bennington	Rural
1940	*Brattleboro	Windham	Rural
	White River Jct.	Windsor	Rural
Post-	*Berlin	Washington	Rural
1940	Springfield	Windsor	

*Hospital-based clinics

The location of pre-1934 clinics for the handicapped in Vermont clearly influenced the location and
nature of the federally co-sponsored CCS clinics.
Unlike Connecticut's emphasis on hospital-based
clinics, Vermont continued its outreach efforts
which pre-existed the federal program. The recollec-
tion of retired health department officials confirm
this interpretation because, for the past 40 years,
Vermont has regularly held clinics in schools and
churches at 13 different locations with a good geographic spread around the state.**

** In addition, weekly clinics were held some years at
Mary Fletcher Hospital in Burlington and in Enosbury
Falls. Also, "plastic" clinics were begun in 1950
in Burlington, Montpelier, Rutland, and Bellow
Falls. The private Caverly Child Health Center was
required under Vermont law to make 30 beds available
to the CCS program in exchange for state funds
(Interview files, Yale Health Policy Project).

for the rural placement of CCS clinics were therefore adequately fulfilled in Vermont.

Clinic location was a very important factor in locating, diagnosing, and treating children with crippling conditions. The availability of service facilities critically affects access and utilization ratios. For instance, in 1939 equal numbers of Connecticut children received CCS services in towns with and without clinics, although towns without clinics had 175,000 more children. The same finding holds for 1969 data despite the two additional hospital-based clinics in the federal-state program. Apparently outreach efforts are unable to compensate for the advantaged access of children living in towns where CCS clinics are located. Hence, Connecticut has only partially fulfilled the rural-oriented goals of the CCS program which Vermont has more adequately achieved.

Job Creation and Professional Beneficiaries

Although partly financed by the federal government, the Title V programs are administered by state governments and are therefore integral parts of each state's administrative system. In order to realize tangible policy goals under the Title V programs, federal government initiatives stimulated changes in personnel practices within state agencies. First through informal recommendations and then by administrative regulations, the federal government required that the new agencies employ medical professionals for program operations. Title V's indirect impacts on state administration in general will be discussed later. Here we focus on historical data about the numbers and professional qualifications of state personnel in Connecticut and Vermont. Despite some limitations on the data due to poor recordkeeping practices and varying classification systems, broad observations can be made about the proportion of health department personnel within each state government, about characteristics of health professionals heading key divisions within the respective health departments, and about the proportion and qualifications of Title V program personnel within each state health department.

In both states, health department personnel generally represent a small fraction of all state employees. When personnel figures for all health-related functions are aggregated in Table X, approximately one-quarter of each state's total employees work in the functional area of 'health'. But this broad category includes state hospital employees, personnel in various specialized but autonomous health agencies, and others not directly controlled by the state health commissioner. A more restrictive criterion of direct administrative jurisdiction over personnel by the health commissioner reveals that no more than one-tenth of Connecticut or Vermont employees ever work for their state's health department. Even comparisons of the latter personnel figures can be misleading because health departments have served at various times as umbrella agencies under which such health-related programs as mental health, mental retardation, tuberculosis hospitals, drug addiction centers, and the like come and go for

Table X: Comparative State Health Personnel (by percent)

Year	All Health Functions		Health Department Only		Total State Employees	
	CT	VT	CT	VT	CT	VT
1950	27		9		(17,448)	
1955	30		8		(20,113)	
1960	29		10		(24,765)	
1965	25	25	10	4	(30,834)	(3886)
1970	22	25	9	5	(45,213)	(5429)
1975		23		4		(6608)

Source: Bjorkman, 1975b.

reasons of administrative convenience. A prime example is the recent relationship in Connecticut between the Office of Public Health and the Office of Mental Retardation. The latter, for want of an institutional home, was assigned to the Health Department during the major governmental reorganization of 1959. During the following decade, the OMR office staff, training schools, and treatment centers grew until they far exceeded their OPH counterparts in size of budget and personnel. Consequently, in 1975 OMR began operations as a full line-department of state government for the same reasons that the mental

health components of Connecticut's health and welfare
agencies were reconstituted into a line-department in
1953.

In any case, whether broadly or narrowly defined,
the proportion of health agency employees in each
state has been basically similar over recent decades.
Given the relative size of its population and personnel pool, Vermont and Connecticut each allocate
equivalent staff resources to health-care operations.
But beyond mere numbers of employees are the qualifications of such employees.

Manpower is vital for any service delivery
system, and professional manpower is critically
important in social policies like education and
health. Professional training in office holders and
their subsequent orientations influence their behavior
as well as the activities of any organization of which
they are a part. Furthermore, professional skills,
values, and knowledge provide links in service
delivery systems that transcend organizational levels
and governmental jurisdictions. Communications
flows among functional specialists cement systems
together.

In Connecticut and Vermont, Table XI reveals a
divergence in the educational credentials of those
who head key divisions in the health department of
each state. In contrast to Vermont's staffing
patterns, Connecticut's upper administrators were
until 1960 more likely to hold doctorates; thereafter
the percentage of bureau heads with doctorates
declined as Connecticut increasingly relied on
personnel with managerial degrees to head its key
divisions. While Connecticut's health department

Table XI: Level of Degrees of the Key Division Personnel
in the Connecticut and Vermont Health Departments
(by percent in educational categories)

Fiscal Year	Doctorates*		Masters**		Bachelors	
	CT	VT	CT	VT	CT	VT
1935-36	46	30	15	20	23	40
1940-41	65	30	6	20	18	40
1945-46	63	46	5	18	21	36

Fiscal Year	Doctorates*		Masters**		Bachelors	
	CT	VT	CT	VT	CT	VT
1950-51	57	50	11	10	11	10
1955-56	61	37	17	20	9	6
1960-61	49	37	22	27	9	5
1965-66	41	55	41	14	10	8
1970-71	40	53	44	5	8	0
1974-75	36	55	50	9	2	0

	No Mention		(Total N)	
	CT	VT	CT	VT
1935-36	15	10	(13)	(10)
1940-41	12	10	(17)	(10)
1945-46	11	0	(19)	(11)
1950-51	11	30	(18)	(20)
1955-56	13	37	(23)	(16)
1960-61	20	32	(45)	(19)
1965-66	8	23	(49)	(22)
1970-71	0	42	(63)	(18)
1974-75	0	12	(58)	(22)

* Includes M.D., D.D.S., L.D., D.V.M.

**Includes M.P.H., R.N., M.B.A.

Source: *Report of the Connecticut Health Department* (1945-46); *Connecticut Health Bulletin* (1947-75); and *Vermont Yearbook* (1928-75).

has recently become more administratively routinized, Vermont's health department has increasingly used physicians in administrative positions. For administrative efficiency, Connecticut seems to have been more rational in managing departmental affairs because officials with modest educational credentials cost less than highly trained experts; in turn, the savings can be used to purchase medical services from the private sector as needed for operating Connecticut's health programs. Vermont, on the other hand, has recently invested more resources in building a highly qualified staff within the health department itself.

However, in the health departments of both states, physicians are in key decision-making positions. Even though Table XII indicates that their proportion is declining in Connecticut as compared to Vermont, those trained in medicine always have a strong plurality and sometimes a clear majority over other health professionals from allied fields like public health, nursing, dentistry, and social work.

Table XII: Professional Training of Key Division Personnel in the Connecticut and Vermont Health Departments (by percent in subject specialty)

Fiscal Year	Medicine*		Public Health		Nursing		Dentistry	
	CT	VT	CT	VT	CT	VT	CT	VT
1935-36	46	30	8	0	8	20	0	0
1940-41	53	30	6	0	6	20	0	0
1945-46	53	46	5	0	6	18	6	0
1950-51	56	50	6	0	6	10	5	0
1955-56	57	37	4	13	4	6	4	0
1960-61	44	31	2	5	2	5	2	5
1965-66	39	43	4	4	2	4	0	4
1970-71	27	43	3	0	2	5	3	5
1974-75	22	47	2	0	2	9	5	4

	Social Work		Other		(Total N)	
	CT	VT	CT	VT	CT	VT
1935-36	0	0	40	50	(13)	(10)
1940-41	0	0	30	50	(17)	(10)
1945-46	0	0	32	36	(19)	(11)
1950-51	0	0	28	40	(18)	(20)
1955-56	0	0	30	44	(23)	(16)
1960-61	0	0	49	54	(45)	(19)
1965-66	2	0	49	45	(49)	(22)
1970-71	2	0	69	47	(63)	(19)
1974-75	2	0	67	45	(58)	(22)

*May include supplementary M.P.H. degree

Source: *Report of the Connecticut Health Department* (1935-46); *Connecticut Health Bulletin* (1947-75); and *Vermont Yearbook* (1928-75).

Degree holders in public health are surprisingly rare
in key administrative positions in both states,
although a number of the physicians have a public
health degree in addition to their medical training.
Interestingly, the importance of non-health training
has increased in both states, and especially in
Connecticut. As hospitals and long-term care
facilities have become increasingly relevant to the
health care system, these 'other' skills have
expanded to include those trained in hospital administration and business management who have been
appointed to responsible administrative positions.

From the first years of Title V operations, the
federal Children's Bureau required that the newly
organized (or recognized) state units be headed by
health professionals. The professional staff was to
develop state-administered programs either by
initiating MCH or CCS de novo or by expanding already
existing efforts. The hired professionals would
serve as intermediaries between federal policy formu-
lators, the service providers in private and/or
public markets, and the program clienteles. Initially,
as the experience of Connecticut reveals in Table
XIII, the bureau responsible for Title V was heavily
staffed with medical professionals. Then, as the
program personnel increased in number, the proportion
of medical professionals declined.

Table XIII: Title V Program Staff in Connecticut's
Bureau of Child Hygiene

	Department Employees	Bureau of Child Hygiene Employees		Medical Professionals Within Bureau of Child Hygiene	
		(N)	Percent	(N)	Percent
1935	112	(14)	13	(7)	50
1938	147	(31)	21	(11)	35
1943	251	(61)	24	(16)	26
1946	342	(100)	29	(16)	16

Source: *Report of the Connecticut Health Department*
(1935-46)

In the Title V operations themselves, the
program staff for MCH and CCS in both states became
a modest proportion of total health department
personnel during the 1940s. Apparently, the share of
program personnel among the total staff of the

department then reached a plateau. Twenty-five years later the proportion of Connecticut's health department staff working on MCH remained relatively unchanged (Friedman, 1974: 75).

In conclusion, if the creation of jobs -- and especially of jobs for professionals -- was another goal of federal child health policy, the historical experiences of Connecticut and Vermont display some supportive evidence. While not necessarily attributable to only Title V initiatives, both state departments of health have expanded and hired many health personnel and particularly physicians. Even in more recent years, when the mix of needed skills diversified, medical doctors have retained their advantage both in relative numbers and in filling key administrative positions.

Chapter IV

Policy Implementation: Indirect Impacts

Intervening Services

In order to link federal initiatives with state
achievements the process of transforming dollars into
deeds was examined. Between fiscal indicators and
the target child populations are several different
service outputs which have been partially financed
with federal dollars. Some services under each
program were directly relevant to health care; others
were only supplementary.

Originally, the Children's Bureau emphasized
direct medical services, clinical examinations of
children, and the establishment of new health clinics.
The Bureau also allowed state programs to purchase
health services from providers on the private market,
thereby subsidizing and reinforcing the classical
pattern of health care delivery. After 1949, however,
regulations began to emphasize such administrative
services as developing standards of quality, delivery
techniques, and personnel training. MCH and CCS
monies could be also increasingly used for overhead
expenses such as salaries and travel costs, rent,
tenant repairs, and upkeep of space exclusively
housing MCH and CCH program units.

Both federal and state funds were increasingly
devoted to these administrative overhead expenses.
During 1953-1959, disbursements for salaries averaged
75 percent of federal-state MCH funds services in
Vermont. Contractual services for health care
constituted another 16 percent of total MCH funds, of
which hospitalization costs absorbed the bulk. The
average share of total CCS funds devoted to salaries
was much lower and averaged 41 percent from 1953 to

41

1972 while contractual services absorbed 51 percent.
Given the nature of the CCS program which financed
both hospitalization and remedial appliances, its
higher average annual disbursements on contractual
services is not surprising. Again hospital costs
represented the single largest expense.

While Title V regulations repeatedly used the
word "services," the content of these services was
not clearly specified. The use of federal funds on
supplemental (non-medical) services did not therefore
contravene the federal statute. Such non-health
services, although difficult to quantify and assess,
must be examined in order to put actual volume of
state-provided health services received by eligible
children into perspective in both states.

The Connecticut MCH program included both direct
and supplementary health services from its origin.
Because the federal Children's Bureau had allowed
state programs to develop, strengthen and improve
standards and techniques, train personnel, and
provide other necessary administrative services,
Connecticut produced a package of multiple MCH
services. The MCH package included well-child
conferences, summer round-ups, inspection, licensing,
consultations, training programs, and site visits,
not all of which are automatically supported by
federal funds. Vermont's package of health services
under MCH appears even more comprehensive; and yet
Vermont apparently spends less on non-health services
like training and inspections than on basic services
like well-child clinics, school health services, and
nursing activities. Nonetheless, as in Connecticut,
site visits and consultations by program personnel
are integral parts of Vermont's MCH activities.

The CCS program is more inclined toward direct
disbursements for child care for it delivers health
care to children through out-patient (clinic, home
or office visits) and inpatient (hospital-based or
in convalescent homes) services. In Connecticut,
only a small percentage of children served ever
actually received inpatient services. As the range
of direct health services became more comprehensive,
the number of inpatients declined. From its minimum
pre-war diagnostic services, the CCS program expanded
to include orthopedic, nephrotic, audial and other
screening and therapeutic services. In addition,
Connecticut also financed advisory, supervisory,

42

and administrative services.

Vermont's CCS activities also reveal elements of an opportunity program. At first, Vermont provided services directly, but now it facilitates their procurement elsewhere. At the same time, Vermont has expanded the range of CCS services. In the early years, orthopedic handicaps were the program's most important priority and that priority remains effective today. But gradually other disease categories were added in the annual State Plans so that Vermont's CCS program emphasized diagnosis, treatment, and post-operative services under six distinct programs (orthopedic; hearing; cleft palate; heart; special services; and chronic disease like cystic fibrosis).

Program personnel provide some of these services directly, but the bulk are purchased through contractual arrangements with private specialists, hospitals, and private agencies for physical therapy, convalescent and rehabilitation care. The independent Caverly Child Health Center, for example, received state financial support in exchange for keeping 30 beds available to the CCS program.

Because the federal government allowed state programs to use federal funds for services not directly related to health, a shift during the forty years of Title V program operations has occurred away from direct health care into supplemental non-health services. This shift occurred earlier, faster and more intensively in Connecticut than in Vermont, but in both states professionals in the MCH and CCS programs spent increasing amounts of time administering the programs instead of delivering services. In this sense, although both states have moved towards programs which putatively expedite opportunities for health care, such shifts in emphasis have been to the detriment of the service programs themselves.

In order to investigate further the proposition that federal policy under Title V also initiated the expansion and maintenance of professional bureaucracies, Title V funds in Vermont were analyzed for their patterns of disbursements. Part of these funds paid salaries and wages to the Vermont State Health Department's central program staff and part financed private health care through purchase of contractual and professional services. Although budgetary materials are often incomplete, manipulated in order to satisfy both federal and state requirements, and tend to lose detailed financial information through the multi-level state reporting process. Vermont's experience from 1937 to 1959 (for MCH) and to 1972 (for CCS) is revealing.

For both Title V programs, "personal services" have reportedly absorbed about 95 percent of the combined federal and state funds since the early 1940s. That rubric consists of three components, namely wages and salaries; contractual services; and professional and consulting services. Most disbursements for contractual services pay hospitalization costs, and most disbursements for professional and consulting services pay medical providers. But for building and sustaining a state bureaucracy, our main interest lies with the proportion of funds used to pay wages and salaries to employees.

Despite some annual fluctuations, Vermont's MCH program clearly reveals a trend toward using its funds to pay wages and salaries to its personnel. Furthermore the allocation of federal funds for such support costs has usually been slightly greater than or at least equal to the allocation of combined funds, which are both in the hands of state officials. As Table XIV indicates, the responsible

Table XIV: Title V Funds Paying Wages and Salaries in Vermont (by percent over five year averages)

Years	Maternal & Child Health		Crippled Children's Services	
	Combined Federal-State	Federal Funds Only	Combined Federal-State	Federal Funds Only
1941-1945	32	36	39	34
1946-1950	53	57	33	32
1951-1955	68	73	41	n.a.
1956-1960	75	75	41	n.a.

Source: *Biennial Report of the Treasurer and Auditor of the State of Vermont*, respective years. Since 1954 periodic changes in the format for reporting fiscal information necessitated using intra-departmental files that were not verified by audits.

federal authorities evidently did not object to this use of funds, which suggests that one impact of federal resources has been to build and strengthen a state bureaucracy.

Unlike MCH, however, the Vermont CCS program displays a more stable, consistent historical record in the use of its funds. Over the decades about two-fifths of combined funds, and an even smaller proportion of federal funds, have been used to finance wage and salary costs; the bulk of the funds, have regularly been paid out for contractual and professional services. Hence, the argument about federal impact on bureaucratic growth of the MCH program cannot be made when analyzing the allocation of CCS monies. Rather than using federal funds for expanding its own administrative infrastructure, Vermont's CCS program has used its funds for purchasing hospital services and professional assistance. Indeed, if any shift has occured in program management, a slightly higher share of state funds since 1955 has gone for personnel support.

But neither state contravened federal policy nor regulations by using its federal funds for supplemental services because federal priorities were never clear. The federal goal of initiating genuine change in child health care was often lost amidst the desires to maintain a system of private health care as well as to establish a professionalized bureaucracy. The professional goals and codes of behavior in turn have reinforced the private health care system which is, after all, operated by the peers of the health professionals in public service.

Patterns of turnover among health officials reveal sharp differences between the two states. The administrative officials responsible for Vermont's MCH and CCS programs change jobs about every five years whereas their Connecticut counterparts demonstrate a remarkable continuity of tenure. Over forty years Connecticut's MCH division has had only four different heads and only two different individuals have headed the CCS program since 1938. The average length of employment for the MCH chief decreases over the forty year history, but former MCH chiefs do not leave the department; they are simply reassigned within it.

Why this marked difference in tenure patterns between the two states? The reason is apparently economic, since salary differentials are substantial between Connecticut and Vermont (U.S. Civil Service Commission, 1963 and 1973). Compared to the private sector, Vermont is clearly at a relative disadvantage in attracting health professionals. Its officials consistently report difficulties in hiring professional personnel because of very low salaries and also in keeping them in their jobs for some time.

State Administration

Indirect effects of federal health policy on both states appeared most markedly in state administration. The respective state assemblies passed conforming legislation in order to meet federal requirements, which produced major innovations in each state's organization set-up. Consonant with its preference for "opportunity policies," the federal government channeled federal dollars toward support functions rather than toward direct health services *per se*. State legislatures and agencies readily accepted these priorities, which simultaneously reinforced the private model of health care and provided ample opportunities for developing professionalized state health bureaucracies.

The Children's Bureau, which administered the MCH and CCS program at the federal level until 1969, influenced the internal structure of each state's executive agencies in several ways. Its interest in the "single agency" concept, an administrative device widespread in New Deal programs that has survived to the present, required that all federal money be channeled through one department. The Bureau expected each designated state agency to exercise complete control and supervision over the state money used for matching purposes. Connecticut's health department did not have such authority, and a change in state law was necessary. Consequently, in 1935, the General Assembly authorized the State Health Commissioner to administer all federal health and welfare funds. In order to qualify for federal funds, the Vermont legislature in a special session likewise immediately gave the State Board of Health an omnibus authorization in a 1935 appropriation bill. Vermont repeatedly renewed this authorization in subsequent appropriation bills until 1947, when

46

the legislature gave the Department of Health
standing authority to receive federal funds whenever
they became available.

Regulations issued by the Children's Bureau also
shaped the internal structure of each department. In
1936, Vermont passed a bill sanctioning federally
initiated organizational changes for maternal and
child health services and services for crippled
children. Public Act No. 10 gave the State Board of
Health broad authority to do anything in its power
to establish the two programs as efficiently and
rapidly as possible. In contrast, Connecticut's
legislature created the two programs directly.

Over the last 40 years, federal interpretation
of the "single agency" concept has changed qualita-
tively. Originally the device required that state
agencies designated to administer federal-state
programs be functional counterparts of the sponsoring
federal agency. Today, the single agency concept is
more comprehensive and relates to the consolidation
of all state agencies receiving federal grants under
one state agency or superagency. Both Connecticut
and Vermont have responded to this trend toward
consolidated reorganization of state agencies.
Vermont brought various departments together under an
Agency of Human Services in 1971 despite opposition
of the health commissioner speaking on behalf of the
State Board of Health. Connecticut tried to create
a single superagency in 1973 and failed.

The practical effects of creating superagencies,
however, seem to have been marginal. Lines of
authority within the Vermont health department and
the Title V programs continue as they did before the
Agency of Human Services was established. One long-
time political activist argues that the only consequence of the reorganized, consolidated agency is
another layer of bureaucracy (Burns, 1972: 8), and
none of our evidence disputes his contention.

One federal bureaucratic requirement has been
lasting. The Children's Bureau required that states
establish separate units for CCS and MCH programs
before federal funds could be released. Although
some states wanted to administer these two programs
jointly, the Children's Bureau maintained its
position until its organizational demise in 1969;
and on July 22, 1974, the *Federal Register* finally

47

allowed the joint administration of MCH and CCS under one program director.

When the Social Security legislation came into effect, Connecticut already had a Bureau of Child Hygiene and thus met the federal requirement for MCH program administration. A new division of Crippled Children, however, had to be created in the Bureau of Child Hygiene in the same year. These separate administrative units have survived, with occasional shifts in nomenclature, the four major administrative reorganizations of the Connecticut State Health Department since the early 30's (Bjorkman, 1975b). Today, both divisions are under the Community Health Services section of the department.

Vermont also made organizational changes to qualify for federal funds. A Bureau of Maternal and Child Hygiene had existed since 1917 but was absorbed by the Division of Public Health Nursing in 1934. In 1936, the Division of Maternal and Child Health was reconstituted to fulfill the requirements of the Social Security Act. Vermont also already had a privately-funded Infantile Paralysis After-Care Division which dated from the 1914 polio epidemic. This agency was brought completely under state control and transformed into the broader Crippled Children Division in 1936. The personnel of the new administrative units, however, were the same as in the two preexisting divisions. Vermont's periodic efforts to obtain federal approval to administer MCH and CCS jointly were opposed by the Regional Office until 1974. At present the Division of Child Health Services remains subdivided into a section on Maternal and Child Health Services, a section on Handicapped Children services, and a section of Child Development Guidance.

Federal regulations not only reshaped state-level administrative structures, but also required state health departments to change their administrative procedures. The Children's Bureau required first the submission of a state plan of action, which was periodically revised. Federal formula funds could only be released after a state's plan had been approved by federal authorities. The plans became increasingly detailed (and confused) over the years, partly because new areas of interest in the health field had developed which required additional decisions, partly because experiences had been gained in program administration, and partly because such lessons had become embedded in the federal regulations.

With each passing decade, the state-level reporting required by the federal government had become more kafkaesque in its complexity. Pressman and Wildavsky (1971) have noted the importance of clearance points for implementing government policies. Originally the Children's Bureau had required state agencies to report both fiscal and service information about child health activities. In order to gain uniform data about health efforts in the American states and about state systems for supervising the actual delivery of services as well as to safeguard federal interests by insuring that states could not easily change or amend their intentions, reports on six different standardized forms had to be submitted. Furthermore, each state plan had to be submitted in triplicate and the quarterly estimates of proposed expenditures had to be submitted in quadruplicate.

Despite the paperwork, the service and fiscal reporting requirements were necessary to insure program accountability. Slowly and surely these reporting requirements expanded and became vehicles for other government policies beyond the narrower conception of child health. For example, since 1935 evidence of compliance with the merit system had to be submitted with state plans. Then in the 1960s, a national concern with civil rights began to penetrate the health-care programs. D/HEW in Washington established a special office for civil rights and ultimately, if Vermont's experience is typical, some 49 individual steps for reporting and clearance were required before a state health plan could be approved (Detore, 1965). More recently, affirmative action has become a federal cause celebre. Such federal goals affect the entire administration of a state's health policy and surface in every individual program. Despite time delays, both Connecticut and Vermont compiled with the multitudinous federal requirements in order to ensure receipt of federal funds.

Fiscal Foibles: An Aside on Financial Practices

Although both states have conformed with federal prescriptions for administering its Title V programs, each has had chronic problems in disbursing its entire annual federal grant. After an audit in 1971, for example, D/HEW sharply criticized the Connecticut State Department of Health for reporting its service and budgetary data late. Between July 1964 and March 1971, some of the mandatory reports had been delayed up to 23 months. The audit also alleged that without seeking interim approval from relevant federal officials, the state agency had used federal funds for services and activities not included in the state plan. Suggestions were made that the Department improve its management and evaluation processes and that its federal funds be better utilized. Table XV shows that during this same period almost one million dollars from the annual grant awards were not disbursed, a situation which reflected adversely on the state's administrative capabilities.

Table XV: Unexpended Funds in Connecticut's Title V Formula Grants, 1965-70

Fiscal Year	Total Award	Funds Not Used	Percentage Not Used
1965	$1,042,277	$150,404	14.4
1966	1,292,074	229,203	17.7
1967	1,460,088	152,972	10.4
1968	1,734,301	214,764	12.4
1969	1,903,324	136,138	7.2
1970	1,917,169	56,525	2.9
Total	$9,349,233	$940,706	

Source: Audit Agency of the D/HEW, Region I, Report on Review of Grants to the State of Connecticut Under Title V of the SSA for the period July 1, 1964 through March 31, 1971, pp. 16-17, file copy.

The fact that state units are incapable of spending all their annual federal funds is not remarkable and indeed is of secondary importance. More significantly, accounting procedures allow the federal government access to state administration and yet federal surveillance of state performance is

decidedly desultory. In response to the federal
allegations, the former State Commissioner of Health
wrote:

"This (auditors) report does not take into
consideration the fact that we are permitted
to rebudget unused Maternal and Child Health
and Crippled Children Fund A in the succeeding
year. Our records show the following:

Fiscal Year	A Funds Rebudgeted
1965	$ 97,548.00
1966	122,960.00
1967	89,666.00
1968	95,016.00
1969	7,624.00
1970	23,142.00
Total	$435,974.00

You will note that the rebudget funds of
$435,974.00 should be subtracted from the
$940,706.00 so the correct amount of funds
which the state*agency did not spend should
be $504,732.00"

The facts available suggest a sympathetic reading of
the Commissioner's explanation for at least half of
the unspent funds. He continued:

Much of our problem stems from lack of
federal direction and uncertainty about
the state plan in recent years. There
seems to have been a change in the federal
approach without finalizing the requirements and providing appropriate interpretation for the states.

Hence federal surveillance of state performance
is inept on two counts. First, it tolerates delays
and whatever program content the state chooses to
sponsor. And second, it misunderstands its own
accounting procedures. Connecticut's poor performance with Title V funds is not excusable but the

_____
*Letter of 10 August 1971 to the Director, Office of
Grants, Management, Health Services and Mental
Health Administration, D/HEW.

federal administrators are equally at fault. The
superficial appearance of regularity and rational
deployment of resources provided by the state plans
is sufficient to satisfy the administrators and to
deter more adequate supervision. While the federal
government has augmented state resources for child
care services and has required large state bureaucracy to meet the multitudinous reporting requirements, it has not been notably successful in ensuring
administrative efficiency.

Vermont's record for fiscal disbursements has
been equally erratic and subject to occasional
federal units. Almost every year from 1936, when MCH
and CCS were first implemented, to 1963 when they
were merged into child Health Services, the Vermont
State Financial Report records an unexpended balance
of state funds for the two programs. And from 1936
to 1955, the Treasurer's Report always reveals an
unexpended balance of their federal funds.* Table
XVI demonstrates that, on the average, more than 20
percent of the annual federal Title V award was not
used. The unexpended state funds "revert to surplus"
which means that they return to the general fund, and
are lost to the MCH and CCS programs. The unexpended
federal funds, however, are deferred for expenditure
during the following fiscal year. State departmental
files indicate that regional audits occurred in 1950
and 1957 but D/HEW's Boston Regional Office was
unable to confirm or deny these audits.

----

*
There are probably unexpended federal MCH and CCS
funds from 1956-63, as well, but these cannot be
identified after 1955 because the federal grants-
in-aid to the health department are *all* lumped together as one entry in the Financial Report.
Furthermore, there may also be unexpended balances
of both federal grants and state appropriations
for the two programs after 1963, but because of
the new system of recording MCH, CCS, and Mental
Health together, separate program records cannot
be extracted.

Table XVI: Unexpended Funds in Vermont

Fiscal Year	Total Award	Funds Not Used	Percent
1936	$ 20,915	$ 1,257	6
1937	35,530	4,509	13
1938	56,610	4,905	9
1939	57,391	8,302	14
1940	75,072	22,759	30
1941	83,185	21,920	26
1942	73,527	19,138	26
1943	82,620	25,007	30
1944	71,697	26,957	38
1945	67,728	24,104	36
1946	65,514*	25,476	39
1947	109,664	33,326	30
1948	115,189	37,625	33
1949	131,983	5,466	4
1950	138,519	18,669	13
1951	157,806	47,716	30
1952	153,776	17,445	11
1953	187,643	26,257	14
1954	151,473	45,121	30
1955	135,139	30,764	23

*Federal expenditure amount used for MCH, because no data on MCH grants for 1946 is available.

Source: Unexpended balances, and MCH and CCS grants for 1936-1946 from *Vermont Biennial Report of Office of Treasurer and Auditor of Accounts;* MCH and CCS grants for 1947-1955 from *Annual Report of U.S. Treasury Office.*

What is curious is that Vermont records both A and B funds as "reappropriated next year". The "A fund" is the flat federal grant-in-aid for Title V operations that goes in equal amounts to each state no matter what its size; the "B fund" is the variable federal grant that is separately calculated for each state according to a formula that considers the number of children, poverty level, and so forth. Federal guidelines stipulate that only A funds may be retained by the states whereas any unexpended B funds must be returned to the federal government. Thus, A funds are always deferred to be tapped only after B funds are spent. It is unclear whether the B funds reported as "reappropriated next year" in the

Vermont Treasurer's Report reflect an error in reporting technique, or a deviation from the federal guidelines. If the latter, perhaps Vermont's chronically late receipt of federal funds persuaded monitoring agents to overlook the discrepancy. Certainly the 'reappropriation' would otherwise have contravened federal practice.

Chapter V

Policy Implementation: Interactive Impacts

State-local relations in Vermont and Connecticut
are similar in that, like other New England states,
both place a high premium on local autonomy.
Connecticut even abolished its counties in 1959
(Levinson, 1966), and Vermont's fourteen counties
have atrophied to the point of serving only as a
convenient classification scheme for recording information. Traditional organization and political
philosophy in these states also reinforce decentralization.

But the Title V programs require centralized
responsibility for decision-making, program
operations, and accountability. The single-agency
concept discussed above, for example, runs counter
to traditional political patterns. Consequently, as
a workable but unwieldy compromise, administrative
and fiscal affairs rest with the state health departments, while service delivery in both states remains
an amalgam of state, local, private, public, and
co-sponsored efforts. Such results alert us to the
impacts of policies on the political system itself,
both when re-inforcing constraints and when changing
opportunities for participation in the policy process.

For example, the pattern of interest group
activity was set early by federal requirements.
Title V monies basically subsidized the prevailing
model of private childcare agencies, professional
medical groups, and other state executive agencies.
Congress itself required states to furnish proof that
they "provide for the cooperation with medical,
health, nursing, and welfare groups and organizations
and with any agency in such state charged with
administering state laws providing for vocational

rehabilitation of physically handicapped children"
(Section 513(a) U.S. Stat. 74th Congress, 1935-1936,
Vol. 49, Part 1, *Public Laws*, p. 623). Both states
immediately obliged by setting up a series of
advisory councils and technical committees. As a
result, medical professionals (in particular
physicians) and health-related groups became well-
entrenched in program administration. Minutes from
committee meetings in Connecticut during the last
'30s reveal a constant concern for the private
sector.

As the Title V programs developed, a network of
institutional relationships encouraged close ties
between governmental health agencies and various
state professional associations. Provider groups
were thus ensured access to health policy process
while the public consumers were generally ignored.
In Connecticut the State Medical Society, the State
Dental Association, the State Nursing Association,
and the Connecticut Branch of the American Association of Medical Workers were all important professional organizations for MCH and CCS program operations. The first and last groups provided the
Health Department with a Technical Medical Advisory
Committee, respectively. Because of overlapping
membership in separate advisory bodies, the influence
of these groups -- and particularly of the Medical
Society -- was cumulative.

Vermont also complied immediately with the
federally-mandated advisory system. In 1935-36 a
State Advisory Committee on Maternal and Child Health
Services was formed which consisted of "physicians,
dentists, and members of lay organizations." In
contrast to Connecticut's practice of including only
established public agencies and recognized professional interest groups, Vermont encouraged some
limited public representation. Linkages between
professional groups and the Title V programs subsequently developed so that official relationships now
exist between the program administrators and the
Vermont State Medical Society, the Vermont Chapter
of the American Academy of Pediatrics, the Vermont
Chapter of the American Academy of General Practice
and the Vermont State Dental Society.

The penetration of professional groups in MCH
and CCS program administration is not unidirectional
either. State program directors occasionally sit on

56

the boards of private associations. For example, the Vermont Director of Child Services serves on the Advisory Board of the Vermont Association for the Crippled, a private association with some public money; she also sits on the School Health Committee and the Welfare Committee of the State Medical Society. Vermont's health commissioner, required by law to be a physician, is expected to belong to the State Medical Society -- although not all Vermont health commissioners have maintained the tie. In turn, the Vermont State Medical Society actively recruits state officials to serve on its committees. Other division directors in the health department, such as the dental section chief, are ex-officio members in their respective professional societies.

The federal policies embedded in Title V also affected political relationships between the branches of government at state-level. Organizational and administrative changes sometimes required conforming legislation and therefore the respective state assemblies up-dated their statutes. State legislatures, however, play only a marginal role in formulating or even over-seeing general health policy, much less child-care policy. Control over the state purse would have been an Assembly's most effective device but the matching funds required by federal law were provided through the health department's annual block appropriations. There was no need to levy special taxes to raise additional revenue.

Put bluntly, knowledge of and concern about child health programs has been limited in legislative circles. In the past 40 years less than one percent of the bills placed before Connecticut's General Assembly's committees have dealt with broadly conceived child-care issues (Bjorkman, 1973a). Indeed, even with generous definitions, only three percent of the Connecticut Assembly's business from 1930 to 1970 was devoted to health and welfare issues. In Vermont the figure was three times greater; but even including issues of environmental health, only ten percent of the 10,904 bills proposed dealt with health and welfare -- and of these, only 332 or about three percent of the total, pertained to children.

The two states also differ on the scope of their public policies for children. Most legislative proposals about health care in Connecticut have been aimed at special target populations with identifiable characteristics. Consonant with the disease-oriented nature of American medical care, preventive measures for the general population have usually been ignored. Most bills proposed in the General Assembly consider those children who are already sick or destitute or abandoned rather than all children; general topics such as child health, maternal health, and school health received little attention whatsoever in the Connecticut legislature. In contrast, Vermont legislators were more likely to consider measures which would apply to all Vermonters. Although a traditional Yankee state characterized by a minimalist philosophy of government, Vermont legislates for the whole rather than for special interests.

Nonetheless, in both states, the legislative assembly plays a minimal role in health affairs. Even the 'oversight' function has been minimized for legislators are more likely to routinely approve decisions in health made elsewhere by administrators and state party leaders (Bjorkman, 1973b). Descriptive studies of the individual federal child-care programs indicate that bureaucrats wield considerable influence in formulating state health policy. Surveys of interest groups have also indicated that lobbyists are less active or at least less visible in the legislative chambers than in administrative corridors. The cumulative evidence suggests that state bureaucrats interact extensively with private interests (Bjorkman, 1974 and 1975b).

Special interest groups affect health care for children, but not always in ways initially expected. One almost axiomatic premise of health-care analysts is that the field is controlled, or at least dominated by, the medical profession. Certainly administrative tables of organization suggest the state medical societies could dominate the policy area because their members sit on a number of advisory boards; the federal regulations also require that these Title V programs have directors who are physicians. Furthermore, physicians in general and pediatricians in particular are patently important providers of health care to children.

Yet medical professionals in both Connecticut and Vermont indicate little concerted activity to implement government programs for child health care. Indeed, the federally-mandated advisory boards are usually moribund; and the activities of medical societies and pediatric chapters are confined to issues of how and how much physicians should be paid for their services in government programs. To be sure, individual physicians contract with state child-health programs in order to diagnose and treat children, but such arrangements are made on an individual basis rather than through the respective professional groups. Thus, while individual doctors have been of critical importance to the success or failure of government programs, doctors as a formally constituted group have not been particularly active in child health.

Why? One reason is that physicians themselves are divided on a host of professional issues. Contrary to lay opinion, all physicians do not have identical interests or compatible views. Some are generalists but most are specialists -- each group with its own more narrowly defined interests. Some physicians practice in rural areas, others in suburbs, still others in cities; each demographic area has its special problems and needs. Also, among practicing physicians, some engage in group practice, but most operate in solo. Other physicians do not engage in private practice at all, but serve hospital staffs, affiliate with teaching hospitals, or engage only in primary research. These various roles, and the forms of financing which underlie them, create strains within state medical societies that are not easily resolved; they also produce internal conflicts that inhibit the medical societies from sustaining much attention in specific government programs.

A second reason for the inactivity of doctors is their conservatism; medical professionals tend to be cautious, resistant to change, and non-innovative. They learn their skills through arduous clinical training and, when applying such received knowledge, tend to become guardians of the status quo. By social definition as well as economic indicators, medical professionals "have it made." Although high social status and economic security need not inhibit the individual physician from acting -- indeed, it is sometimes argued that status and security allow the individual to take risks -- spokesmen for those with

59

high status and economic security seek to maintain
their dominance over the contemporary order of things.
They have, as one critic argues, "structural
interests" in the contemporary health-care system
as it exists (Alford, 1974).

Third, many professional groups outside the
national capital are not well organized for continual
involvement in the policy process. State medical
societies are sometimes an exception to the rule,
but often even their internal committees are organi-
zationally episodic. If annual reports of the Vermont
and Connecticut medical societies are accurate, only
a minimal staff is supported by the dues-paying
members and each staff tends to pursue narrowly
defined professional activities. Medical professionals are understandably preoccupied with their private
practices or with their own relationships to
hospitals, insurance companies, and regulatory
agencies; but as a consequence, they are only
marginally involved, if at all, with public policy
affairs in Connecticut and Vermont.

While internal conflict, innate conservatism,
and inadequate organization characterize most groups
of professionals, one should not infer the absence
of professional influence on public policy decisions.
But such professional influence is the product of
individual motivation and effort rather than the
product of group inspiration and direction. A
physician who heads the child-health program in a
state health department and who also serves as
liaison to the medical society's standing committee
on maternal and child health -- such a person can be
crucial for the success of a program. Unfortunately
in the historical sweep of our investigations, such
individuals are the exception rather than the rule.

The American public usually regards health
affairs -- and even more so child-health affairs --
to be the responsibility of medical experts with
specialized training. Given the minimal amount of
self-help and self-care in health, the triumph of
'professionalism' as a public ideology can be termed
an almost total 'civic religion'. Even at a public
level, politicians defer to health statesmen; and
when health statesmen are primarily defined to be
medical professionals, their policy recommendations
incline toward conservative, status-quo solutions
(Dalston, no date). In short, as Vermont and

Connecticut bear witness, medical professionals
supply irresolute support for public child health
programs.

If professional interests are generally inactive
in Title V's child-health programs, what about other
spokesmen for children? Does anyone speak for the
'health interests' of children? Before examining the
historical record in Connecticut and Vermont, we
should mention some problems that confront anyone
advocating better services for children, whether such
services be educational, recreational, or physical.
Stated simply, about forty percent of the American
population are less than twenty years old, and that
enormous demographic category is just too large, too
amorphous, and too internally varied to be easily
organized. "Children" range from infants through
adolescents to young, physically mature adults -- and
each age-span has its own unique problems. In
contrast, the elderly are much more homogeneous in
problems and needs, and subsequently are easier to
organize (Vinyard, 1976). Furthermore, except for
the career professionals discussed above, advocates
of child health services are transients; that is,
even parents anticipate the day when their children,
grown to adulthood, no longer draw upon family
resources (Kenniston, 1974: 10). Arguably, a
'rational' parent prefers short-run investments to
long-run financial commitments--although obvious
exceptions exist when offspring with congenital or
accidental defects will never be able to cope for
themselves. Consequently, the large numbers,
diversity, and transitory status of those who could
potentially be organized to promote the health of
children mean that child health advocates have three
strikes against them before they even begin to bat.

Nonetheless, caveats aside, there are advocates
for child health in the two states. And yet another
political impact of federal initiatives has been the
incentives which they provide for a group to
organize. Decisions about diagnostic categories for
CCS treatment, for example, had been left to the
states. In Connecticut, several groups therefore
formed at state level to lobby for access to Title V
programs. Usually state health administrators
exercised their discretion to include new clients
whenever possible, but in several cases the costs of
providing such additional treatment would have been
prohibitive. The state agency then declined, usually

regretfully, to expand its roles. In turn groups of
parents organized in order to press their claims in
the public and legislative arenas. Advances in
medical technology facilitated their efforts because
new methods of treatment became available.

To mention but a few diseases, associations were
formed on behalf of those children afflicted with
cystic fibrosis, cerebral palsy, and cardiac defects.
In 1947, in 1950, and again in 1955 the Connecticut
General Assembly passed legislation to include
rheumatic heart disease, cerebral palsy, and cystic
fibrosis, respectively, in the state's CCS program.
Connecticut's CCS director credits these special
legislative enactments to the activities of
interested parents' groups. While other interest
groups often express the fear of looking 'political',
the object lessons provided by the Parents Association of Cardiac Children, by the United Cerebral
Palsy Association, and by the Cystic Fibrosis
Association of Connecticut are clear.

Vermont, to the contrary, has no record of
extensive activity by such special-interest consumer
groups. Perhaps the reason for this lacuna is
Vermont's small population. It lacks the critical
mass to generate enough special cases that could
then, in turn, organize in order to extract special
treatment from the state. In recent years, a novel
force for progressive health legislation in Vermont
has emerged. The consumer-oriented Vermont Public
Interest Research Group has adopted child-care as
one of its many worthwhile causes (Peterson, 1975).
The Connecticut counterpart to this omnibus consumer
lobby has been conspicuously less active in broad
social policies.

Another reason for the relative absence of
special-action groups in Vermont's health politics
is that state's tendency to require its bureaucracy
to treat all citizens on an equal footing. If, as
an example, the financial impossibilities for a
family with a hemophiliac child were brought to the
legislature's attention, it would (and did) mandate
the health department to provide hemophiliac families
with needed care. It did not, however, vote
additional funds but left the department to manu-
facture the needed skills from its internal
resources. A more salient, and well-funded, case is
that of Vermont's "Tooth Fairy" program which

broadened eligibility criteria of the federal Denti-
caid program and added state funds so that all
Vermont children obtained dental examinations and,
as necessary, subsidized dental treatment.

In addition to groups of providers and consumers
of child-health services in the two states, another
category of relevant actors are those who collect and
disburse the funds for health services. Exclusively
focusing on federal and state funds in Title V operations produces an incomplete picture of federal
impacts. The prevailing pattern of funding arrangements is, in many ways, an even more important "non-
decision" of federal policy-makers than their
"decision" to provide Title V funds. That is, while
various levels of government directly control
finances in other social policies such as education,
in health care most money flows completely within the
private sector through third-party payors like
insurance companies. Fiscal intermediaries other
than government agencies have resources, organization, and skills to influence public policy. But
even if chartered as nonprofit corporations, insurance companies are more concerned with efficient
operations than with the health status of children.

Furthermore, the insurance industry is one of
the largest business activities still regulated
primarily by state governments, and such state-level
regulation in fifty separate jurisdictions is pre-
ferred by the insurance companies themselves. In
1944, the U.S. Supreme Court extended federal jurisdiction over insurance companies by broadly inter-
preting the Constitution's clause on interstate
commerce, but Congress expressly voted in 1945 to
delegate responsibility for regulating insurance to
the states. Barring certain evident exceptions,
regulatory authority over insurance remains at state
level (Krizay and Wilson, 1974: 43).

Since state governments put up part of the cost
of health care through matching funds, the state
governments through their insurance commissioners try
to exert pressure on fiscal intermediaries to keep
costs down and administrative overheads low. The
Vermont State Insurance Commissioner has kept Blue
Cross and Blue Shield under very tight rein by
systematically rejecting or diminishing their proposals for increases in premium rates. Unsurprisingly,
spokesmen for the Blues have been concerned about

issues other than their ability to influence state child-health policy.

Although not as salient nor as powerful as insurance companies, private nonprofit voluntary associations like The Society for Crippled Children and Adults (Easter Seals) also collect and disburse funds for health care. As the nation has moved incrementally toward a public welfare state, the philanthropic role of Easter Seals has declined but in the relatively restricted field of child health programs, Easter Seal affiliates finance many services for the chronically handicapped. These services range from case finding to amelioration to curative efforts and rehabilitation. Nonetheless the Easter Seal organizations in Connecticut and Vermont focus on relatively restricted programs and consequently do not provide the leadership needed for an overall, coordinated health policy for children. Limited resources and personnel plus an insecure financial future cause Easter Seal Societies to confine themselves to standard, routine activities. And indeed, a repeatedly expressed fear among Easter Seal administrators is that the era of the voluntary philanthropic organization will soon be over because state and federal governments are moving into their baliwick of specialized social services in a major, sustained way.

To summarize the 'group scene' after forty years of federal impacts on child-health in Connecticut and Vermont, it is quiescent. Traditional health providers are passive; health consumers are organized, when at all, into "hit-and-run" associations with very specialized needs; and fiscal intermediaries have other issues to pursue. At times marginal changes have occured, but the entire system demonstrates great continuity with the prevailing situation in the 1930s.

64

Chapter VI

Implications for Social Policies

What lessons, then, can be drawn from the performance of these two New England states over the past four decades? There are some obvious findings that Vermont does a better job of utilizing federal Title V programs than does Connecticut although neither is outstanding. But in addition to conclusions about their comparative track records in child health care, are there any features of politics or administrative organization that associate with the implementation and impact of federal-state programs in our intergovernmental system? And what are the effects of financing mechanisms on the provision of health care? The two states are sufficiently disparate to allow us to conclude that any similarities between them may be generalizable to other states. And any differences may suggest propositions for investigation elsewhere.

We should emphasize that our primary interests lie with the analysis of public policy as procedure rather than with the substantive analysis of children's health. Thus we have examined political and administrative factors instead of the conditions of health care. But the quest for better child health care is a representative social policy that provides a typical set of constraints and parameters for action. A broad-gauge goal like improving child health is sufficiently amorphous to admit many interpretations. And while ambiguous federal goals hamper the evaluation of social policies' implementation and impact, they allow a wide latitude for flexible response to political needs.

Ambiguous as health policy may be, however, both
Connecticut and Vermont demonstrate more continuity
than change in their health care provisions for
children. The continuity is more one of neglect than
nurture because child-health is not a subject that
claims much attention in state politics. And although
children comprise some two-fifths of the whole population, child health is usually considered in terms of
remedial or corrective measures rather than preventive ones. Only some three percent of government-
financed health expenditures go into preventive
programs; the balance goes into treatment, rehabilitation, and administration. The advantages of an
emphasis on remedial treatment for the provider
interests is obvious for their livelihood is bound up
in the provision of direct care. The consumer-
citizen, although perhaps individually aware that an
ounce of prevention is worth a pound of cure, does not
push for a 'forward' policy of preventive health with
its demonstrable savings. But given the American
health care system, such as it is, it may be important
to consider improvements in case-finding and treatment
even before lamenting the low salience of preventive
health policies.

Initial investigations in Connecticut indicated
that federal initiatives did not increase state
attentiveness to the conditions of child health.
Indeed, if anything, the Title V funds just supplemented and partially supplanted the pre-existing state
program for maternal and child hygiene. The same
argument applies to Vermont which had a state-financed
program since 1917 for all Vermonters afflicted with
infantile paralysis, only to restrict eligibility by
age when the CCS program was instituted in 1935.

In more recent years, Vermont has demonstrated
the type of stimulative effect that the classical
American federal theory about pump-priming would
expect. After Medicaid provided federal-state funds
for dental care for welfare children, the state
enacted and implemented a "tooth fairy" bill which
provided a graded scale of partial payments for all
Vermont children. At present, guided by the example
of EPSDT which can if implemented provide welfare
children with comprehensive health care, the Vermont
legislature is also considering a parallel bill that
would extend comparable benefits to all children in
the state. The federal example has been accepted and
elaborated, thus justifying a standard argument for

federal aid: help the states to help themselves.

It is not clear, however, whether maximum payoff from federal funds comes from financing expansion of the bureaucracy, underwriting through third-party payments the provision of health care by private physicians, or paying physicians directly as the Veterans Administration already does. Each investment route has its benefits and drawbacks, and the subject needs further exploration and research. But given the relatively poor performance record for child-health services in these two states, it may be advisable to use more dollars for direct services than for overhead costs. At present, more than half of all program funds go into administrative salaries and contractual expenses rather than into direct health services.

The question again is what federal policy for child health intends to achieve. In the initial years of Title V, when the well-being of both providers and consumers was jeopardized by an economic depression, services tended to provide medical and health care directly. Since then, there has been a trend toward facilitating services to replace direct services in federal-state health programs. As the policy of providing opportunities rather than direct care increased, the status quo was reinforced. The full consequences of this shift toward administrative expansion on the condition of child health in the states examined is unclear because no baseline of health-care needs exists against which the relative gap of unmet need can be measured and assessed. But it seems fairly obvious that 'opportunity' policies support pre-existing patterns of society in addition to adding members to the facilitating bureaucracy. And since the United States already had a commitment to the market economy and a network of private providers of health care was already in place, the federal-state programs were developed in such a way as not to threaten their basic interests. Further research is clearly necessary as to how the distribution of financial resources connects with changes in health status.

Because of the elastic tax-base of the federal government and because the provision of funds is a major federal level over state policies, further research into funding patterns is also advisable. But the experiences of Connecticut and Vermont with the formula funds provided under Title V programs indicates that the states were left free to do as they wished. While centralization and standardization are often high priorities on the agendas of both presidential administrations and the permanent federal bureaucracies, the mechanism of formula funds has been favored by the US Congress which is more prone to defend states' rights than to centralize government. Consequently, despite the superficial appearance that states must conform with federal requirements before obtaining their formula funds, formula grants became a prototype for revenue sharing.

In point of fact, the states are permitted by federal officials to meet the legal and regulatory requirements of matching federal funds with state resources through such easy methods as allowing matching funds in-kind rather than in-cash. As long as the superficial 'form' was maintained, the substantive content and impact of Title V programs did not greatly matter. Indeed, one of the chief selling-points for the formula-fund mechanism was that it took account of local conditions rather than imposing a centralized standard on all areas, and the state plans approved by federal monitoring officials varied enormously.

Some of the more valuable lessons from Connecticut and Vermont about the impact of intergovernmental programs lies in the fields of politics and administrative organization. The political lessons may verge upon tautological arguments because policy is in fact politics in concrete, substantive form. And a cautionary note is that a pair of cases from one region of the United States provides an inadequate basis for extensive generalizations. But the comparative case-studies do reveal features of the domestic policy-process which merit further exploration.

In very general terms, the thesis is provocative that a small state can attain a better performance record than a larger state. Large size is usually associated with the critically needed resource base to implement programs because without some resources in tax dollars and infrastructure, nothing can be accomplished. Yet small size seems to be associated with efficiency, thorough processing of information, accountability, and manageability. The economics of scale may be off-set and negated by the handicaps of

68

excessive size and complexity. These effects of size on quality-control, innovativeness, risk-taking, and support need further research and analysis.

Acknowledging the limitations of a two-state sample, it also appears that objective resources and characteristics of states are insufficient predictors of policy outcomes. Vermont has the better record in child-health programs, yet Connecticut is the wealthier, more progressive, urbanized, and industrialized state. With such excellent resources at the disposal of its policy-makers and administrators, one would expect that Connecticut's performance would surpass that of most states. But such is not the case, and one explores reasons why.

Perhaps the better program performance in Vermont is a consequence of its rural nature and the needs of its politicians to meet the needs and expectations of its rural areas where most of the voters reside. An urban, industrialized state is more likely to shortchange its rural sector because the latter has less power than urban constituencies. Title V programs were, and still are, directed at "rural and economically depressed areas." And certainly as measured by activity in the legislatures, child-health gets three times as much consideration in Vermont as in Connecticut. Furthermore, Vermont stresses the general condition of child-health while Connecticut focusses on special target populations. The more highly specialized, differentiated nature of an urban state may be the cause of this 'hit and run' tactic of health-care legislation since urban groups see themselves in competition with other groups for scarce resources.

In general we found that policy goals vary sharply between the two states. Legislative goals in Vermont are universal in scope; in Connecticut they are more restrictedly specific to special interests. In Vermont, interest groups are less specialized and fewer in number than in Connecticut; they are also less active. Admittedly the topic for this interstate comparison has been restricted to child health. But Vermont has produced the more progressive legislation despite our initial expectation that liberal Connecticut would have a much better track record. Unlike Connecticut's emphasis on physical treatments which favor selected groups, Vermont's theme has been a concern for the general well-being of all, if such were fiscally feasible.

This contrast in legislative orientations and group activities is repeated in the respective administrative programs for child health. Vermont has emphasized total child's care from screening for initial crippling symptoms to rehabilitative education and special compensatory social skills. Unlike Connecticut's stress on curative and ameliorative mechanisms, Vermont's programs touch on both preventive and restoration.

Why Connecticut and Vermont diverge so sharply is puzzling, and the finding contravenes some conventional wisdom. Knowledge that Vermont has a history of domination by the Republicans or that Connecticut is a swing-state with Democratic proclivities does not produce very meaningful predictions. And the greater, more extensive activity by groups in Connecticut did not lead to more or better distributed health care. In other words, the overt political inputs like party domination and group activity do not relate directly to the scope and impact of health policy--unless we should conclude that GOP philosophy more generally favors a comprehensive commonweal and that excessive group participation in politics leads to pernicious effects. The latter may well be true if the enlarged arena of competing groups produces a 'hit-and-run' philosophy of politics which seeks to extract whatever is possible from the state without cooperating with other groups. In neither state, however, can it be said that health policy derives from interest group activity any more than it does from any other single factors. At least on the issue of child health care, the presumed significance of interest groups is much over-rated.

If the political factors in making and implementing policy for child health in the intergovernmental system are puzzling, the lessons about the bureaucracy are more clear. Many of the outcomes appear to trace back to the politics of the bureaucracy and the standard arguments of incremental decision-making. Like policy activists, policy analysts tend to think in simplistic terms and we often assume that the federal government, or a state government, is a single monolithic entity. The truth, in fact, is that governments are congeries of multiple units; and these units within even a single level of government can play multiple, sometimes contradictory, roles. Thus, for example, the federal agencies responsible for the condition of children's health in the United States can both initiate and squelch measures on their behalf. An agency can be both initiator and depressant. Furthermore, the bureaucratic competition within one level of government is as important to understand as the interrelationships between levels of government.

For example, when lamenting the lack of long-term planning and assessments of past efforts, we cannot underemphasize the short-run nature of most decision-making. Participants in both Congress and the legislatures, in the federal bureaucracy and state administrations, seek marginal benefits to their current situations. Politicians most often want to be re-elected; bureaucrats want to maintain, and sometimes expand, their agencies. In sum, the most basic motivation for all players in the system is the advancement or continuation of their private careers. Democratic pluralism seeks to reconcile and bury conflicts rather than revealing and sharpening them; hence log-rolling and favor-trading by both politicians and bureaucrats are likely forms of behavior. Consequently, when an investigator seeks to evaluate the impact of a particular program or policy, he asks the wrong questions unless he begins with the hidden agendas of the participants.

One continuous drawback of our own research has been the obvious inadequacy of the documentary and service data for assessing the direct impact of Title V programs. It is repeatedly frustrating to find that reporting requirements, like planning requirements, tend to camouflage more than they reveal. The only criterion of relevance that applies is that the prestructured reporting or planning forms devised in Washington or the regional offices be completely filled out. Yet because the state and local data varied so extensively, the result of such forms has been procrustean; they distorted more than they reported. Hence the data are not comparable, although such appears to be the case. In fiscal data, for example, administrative accounting and reporting devices or conventions wreak havoc with attempts to establish the actual share of expenditures (in-cash or in-kind) provided by respective state and federal sources. Ironically, the final consequence may well have been the initial intent,

namely to mask responsibility and prevent direct
accountability.

The hypothesized importance of personnel on
program performance is less clear. Although tentative, the pattern of increasing the educational qualifications of bureaucrats and of adding professional
specialists does not appear to have had a notable
impact. Neither is it clear that as a ratio of all
bureaucrats, the numbers of professionals have
increased. It is, however, true that in absolute
numbers in both states there are more health professionals in top staff positions today than forty years
ago, and hence these professionals man the commanding
heights of state efforts at public health care.
Control of strategic positions may be more crucial
than numerical domination, since such control provides
an easy access-route to the bureaucrat's professional
peers in the private world of medical specialists.
In quantitative terms, the health professionals
benefit less from the creation of additional bureaucratic jobs than we had anticipated; but in qualitative terms, the health professions were probably
well served by the expanding bureaucracy.

The findings on tenure and turnover of bureaucrats in health care agencies and programs are ambiguous and almost contradictory, depending on the
level of appointment. Program heads in Vermont are
replaced frequently while in Connecticut they remain
for many years. Given the comparative performance
records, we might conclude that tenure has had a
depressing effect on accomplishments; or put alterna-
tively, that frequent turnover loosens up the system
and promotes better implementation of program goals.
But at the departmental level, the commissioners in
both states have served very long terms of office.
The post of chief public health officer has been
considered an a-political one worthy of bi-partisan
support since public health is a universal concern.
Nonetheless in one state, the health department's
share of total budget outlays declined while it
increased in the other. Another area to explore,
then, is the role of leadership per se and the skills
which leaders bring to bear on situations. Leaders
of course may be administrators as well as politicians, and such research should include investigations
of the governors' offices as well as departmental
and program heads.

A final conclusion about the bureaucracy emerges
from the historical experiences of both states.
Organization theory argues that structural changes
affect the quality and performance of an agency's
functions. And federal policy, both in money and
standards, undoubtedly changed the shape and size
of state-level administration. More personnel were
added; specialized division of labor occured; coor-
dination between the private and public sectors
became more necessary. But it is difficult to disen-
tangle the 'natural growth' of an expanding state
economy from the 'induced growth' of federal impacts,
especially in health care. It can be argued, in
fact, that federal health monies have a substitutive
rather than stimulating effect on state expenditures;
rather than stimulating a state to generate more
funds earmarked for health programs, the federal
grants-in-aid for health only released state tax-
resources for use elsewhere. In any case, these
trends, although not directly traceable to federal
initiatives, make the policy-goals of improving the
health of children simultaneously easier and more
difficult to achieve.

In sum, the lessons from Connecticut and Vermont
are not startling. If anything, they are instead
sobering and temper the grand rhetoric that appeared
in the Congressional mandate some forth years ago.
Federal efforts under Title V do not lessen the
general neglect of child-health measures in state
legislation. Nor have they greatly expanded the
volume of direct services for child-care beyond those
already existing before 1935. Federal efforts are,
however, sufficiently ambiguous and diffuse to leave
the providers dominant in treating diseases and
conditions that already exist rather than focussing
energy and attention on preventive health measures.
Federal efforts, in short, reinforce the prevailing
system of private health care because federal
resources are absorbed by the costs of expanding
administrative overhead. Yet these federal efforts
inflate rather than greatly influence state bureaucracies. And as a consequence, continuity rather
than change appears to be the more lasting impact
of federal initiatives in the health care system.

73

Appendix A

PRIMARY DATA

Table 1: Maternal and Child Health

Year	Federal Grants[1] Current	Federal Grants[1] Constant*	Federal Expenditures[2] Current	Federal Expenditures[2] Constant*	Total Expenditures[2] Current	Total Expenditures[2] Constant*	Number of Children[3]
1936	31,034	72,679					7,990
1937	41,223	92,636					8,445
1938	37,281	84,923					10,087
1939	52,074	120,542					5,656
1940	65,322	148,797			95,151	216,893	6,907
1941	70,632	149,644			107,730	228,145	6,705
1942	55,320	104,377			106,732	201,267	9,878
1943	58,395	102,808			105,291	185,274	
1944	57,539	98,884			114,332	196,582	9,693
1945	64,800	108,543			120,075	201,266	4,431
1946	80,860	121,229			124,734	187,008	8,363
1947	171,776	230,262			180,126	241,326	3,808
1948	85,585	107,591			191,529	240,831	4,119
1949	100,925	127,592			209,062	260,442	4,250
1950	97,434	121,489			211,855	264,290	5,039
1951	117,096	136,794			198,978	232,342	5,347
1952	119,064	136,073					5,022
1953	142,484	161,364					
1954	124,300	138,728			215,082	239,967	6,716
1955	130,314	143,360			212,425	233,794	5,151
1956	144,763	154,003					4,821
1957	214,271	219,765					6,623
1958	257,922	257,922					3,955
1959	246,266	242,388					3,257
1960	259,346	251,081					3,424

Year	Federal Grants [1]		Federal Expenditures [2]		Total Expenditures [2]		Number of Children [3]
	Current	Constant*	Current	Constant*	Current	Constant*	
1961	282,749	270,315	279,770	264,483	557,986	527,497	3,160
1962	356,556	337,073	311,033	290,224	573,671	535,290	3,083
1963	329,747	307,836	345,270	317,198	700,380	643,987	2,593
1964	382,737	351,610	401,608	331,231	1,026,787	926,202	2,434
1965	445,223	401,608	502,999	469,955	999,914	877,579	2,451
1966	573,117	502,999	585,002	439,231	819,530	596,981	2,173
1967	687,904	585,002	589,454	419,330	1,061,117	827,704	2,264
1968	720,902	589,454	510,298	670,569			2,523
1970	690,127	510,298	570,132				2,410
1971	807,307	570,132					

Appendix A: Primary Data on Connecticut

Table 2: Crippled Children's Services

Year	Federal Grants[1]		Federal Expenditures[2]		Total Expenditures[2]		Number of Children[4]
	Current	Constant*	Current	Constant*	Current	Constant	
1936							314
1937							667
1938	33,735	76,845					965
1939	17,977	41,613					1,121
1940	31,671	72,144			78,810	179,664	1,367
1941	67,641	143,307			80,007	169,435	1,486
1942	75,453	142,364			98,518	185,966	1,768
1943	33,693	59,319			94,486	166,260	2,129
1944	72,458	124,498			114,927	162,459	2,245
1945	79,345	132,906			132,929	222,811	2,535
1946	68,206	102,258			130,350	195,427	2,848
1947	143,731	192,669			150,714	201,921	3,592
1948	86,245	108,348			167,537	210,553	3,521
1949	131,456	166,190			161,820	261,170	2,989
1950	134,837	168,126			206,368	257,445	2,859
1951	179,000	209,112			190,136	220,018	2,968
1952	177,200	202,514					2,924
1953	175,768	199,058					2,911
1954	182,906	204,136			275,972	307,901	2,975
1955	191,172	210,310			288,680	317,720	3,037
1956	211,683	225,195					
1957	216,950	222,513					
1958	214,457	214,457					
1959	213,640	210,276					4,390
1960	221,340	214,269					3,642

78

Table 2: Crippled Children's Services (Continued)

Year	Federal Grants[1]		Federal Expenditures[2]		Total Expenditures		Number of Children[4]
	Current	Constant*	Current	Constant*	Current	Constant	
1961	257,068	245,763	208,583	197,185	414,958	392,284	3,100
1962	286,180	270,491	317,408	296,172	966,367	901,462	2,756
1963	301,310	281,073	317,115	291,332	574,750	527,778	3,893
1964	302,024	277,596	283,257	255,509	655,910	591,443	4,098
1965	353,990	319,197	395,197	346,847	777,106	683,270	
1966	384,907	337,934	412,383	350,969	905,538	770,015	
1967	443,813	377,392	323,888	264,831	764,668	525,240	4,000
1968	447,555	385,948	409,704	319,582	925,971	722,286	3,200
1969	502,313	321,899	418,608	390,530	843,042	623,552	3,200
1970	512,098	378,770					
1971	528,134	372,976					
1972	531,100	363,518					

Appendix A: Sources for Primary Data on Connecticut

*Source of the implicit price deflator (1958=100) is the Department of Commerce, Bureau of Economic Analysis.

[1]Data source 1936 through 1956 is *Report of Comptroller, Connecticut Public Documents,* respective years. Data source 1956 through 1970 is *Annual Report of the United States Secretary of the Treasury,* respective years. Grants for mental retardation programs have been excluded from MCH figures, as have grants for special M & I and C & Y projects. Also, grants are recorded only in the year of their initial award; annual figures do not include any carry-overs of unspent funds. Thus, an annual federal expenditure may logically exceed an annual federal grant.

[2]Data source 1940 through 1955 is "Detailed Expenditures of All Funds." *Report of the Comptroller, Connecticut Public Documents,* respective years. Data source 1962 through 1970 are "Quarterly Statement of Recipients and Expenditures of Federal Funds for Health Services" and "Quarterly Statement of Grant Awards and Expenditures of Federal Funds for MCH and/or SOC," D/HEW. Expenditures on mental retardation programs have been excluded, as have expenditures for special M & I and C & Y projects.

[3]Data source 1923 through 1946 is *Department of Health Annual Report,* respective years. Data source 1947 through 1972 is *Annual Administrative Report to the Governor,* respective years. Supplementary data sources are "MCH Health Services Provided or Paid for by State or Local Official Public Health Agencies," respective years from 1946 through 1970, published by the Children's Bureau in Washington, D.C.; MCH Statistical Series, respective years from 1955 through 1970; and Health Policy Project files. Through 1946, the number of MCH children treated include those covered in the Summer Round-Up program. Thereafter, only children seen at state co-sponsored Well-Child Conferences are recorded.

[4]Data source 1938 through 1952 is *Connecticut Health Bulletin,* 68: 3 (March 1954): 114. Data source 1947 through 1972 is *Annual Administrative Report to the Governor,* respective years.

Appendix A: Primary Data on Vermont

Table 3:   Maternal and Child Health

Year	Federal Grants[5]		Federal Expenditures[6]		Total Expenditures[7]		Number of Children[9]
	Current	Constant	Current	Constant	Current	Constant	
1937	23,313	52,984	16,620	37,773	19,601	44,548	
1938	36,377	82,675	35,736	81,218	45,538	103,498	
1939	38,981	90,653	36,187	84,156	46,339	107,765	
1940	57,774	131,304	43,809	99,566	58,025	131,875	
1941	60,115	127,904	60,408	128,528	74,376	158,247	
1942	48,337	91,277	55,128	104,015	80,768	152,393	
1943	61,649	108,156	58,279	102,244	77,305	135,623	
1944	50,722	87,452	49,850	85,948	69,179	119,274	
1945	51,812	86,353	49,320	82,200	67,467	112,445	
1946			42,145	62,903	64,091	95,658	
1947	74,450	99,267	66,771	89,028			
1948	69,652	87,065	71,579	89,474			
1949	53,811	68,115	69,566	100,716	130,844	165,625	
1950	72,895	91,119	58,315	72,894			
1951	80,601	93,722	67,954	79,016			
1952	76,571	88,013	102,346	114,995	142,874	164,223	
1953	87,615	99,562	84,069	95,533	133,816	152,064	
1954	78,760	87,511	65,727	72,227	136,918	152,131	
1955	71,102	78,134	86,386	93,831	156,330	171,791	
1956	77,007	81,922	77,224	82,153	159,299	169,467	33,943
1957	100,313	103,415	90,543	93,343	171,507	176,811	32,056
1958	105,640	105,640	102,953	102,953	187,688	187,688	31,256
1959	107,217	105,115	100,821	99,823	198,043	194,160	29,836
1960	109,734	106,538	100,876	97,938	194,936	189,258	33,506

Table 3: Maternal and Child Health (Continued)

Year	Federal Grants[5]		Federal Expenditures[6]		Total Expenditures[7]		Number of Children[9]
	Current	Constant	Current	Constant	Current	Constant	
1961	120,184	114,461	114,975	109,500	205,689	195,894	31,271
1962	125,742	118,624	117,365	110,722	224,446	209,763	37,577
1963	138,721	120,300	128,026	119,650	240,607	224,866	29,210
1964	135,169	124,008	125,775	115,390			31,129
1965	137,635	123,995					17,136
1966	166,738	146,261	161,013	141,239	267,118	240,647	31,685
1967	177,114	150,097					23,502
1968	177,663	145,625	175,707	144,022	298,236	252,742	21,786
1969	177,686	138,738					23,461
1970	136,000	100,740	136,000	100,741	340,540	266,047	22,977
1971	290,921	204,874	294,312	207,261			32,098
1972	195,331	133,788	137,965	94,497			32,103
1973	205,772	133,618			439,203	300,824	20,915
1974	274,243						

Appendix A: Primary Data on Vermont

Table 4: Crippled Children's Services

| Year | Federal Grants [5] | | Federal Expenditures [6] | | Total Expenditures [8] | | Number of Children [9] |
	Current	Constant	Current	Constant	Current	Constant	
1937	12,217	27,766	15,753	35,802	33,756	78,718	
1938	19,233	43,711	20,051	45,570	46,485	82,920	
1939	18,410	42,814	17,965	41,179	37,165	86,430	
1940	17,298	39,314	16,846	38,286	35,778	81,314	
1941	23,070	43,528	23,017	48,972	41,860	89,064	
1942	25,150	47,452	21,563	40,685	41,559	78,413	
1943	20,971	36,789	19,841	34,809	29,385	69,096	
1944	20,975	36,164	19,429	33,498	39,164	67,559	
1945	15,916	26,527	20,440	34,067	40,380	67,300	
1946	23,369	34,879	26,741	39,912	44,923	67,049	
1947	35,214	36,952	35,042	46,723			1,421
1948	45,537	56,921	39,312	49,140			1,622
1949	52,417	66,351	58,622	74,205	91,614	115,967	1,549
1950	65,624	82,030	66,612	83,265	76,612	95,765	1,670
1951	77,205	89,773	65,375	76,017			1,753
1952	72,972	83,876	72,896	83,788	124,331	142,909	1,954
1953	100,028	113,668	94,763	107,685	150,227	170,712	2,134
1954	72,713	80,792	65,881	74,312	127,011	141,123	2,240
1955	64,037	70,370	82,459	90,614	149,633	164,432	2,264
1956	97,606	103,836	95,647	101,752	164,413	174,907	2,330
1957	97,263	100,271	84,255	86,861	161,523	166,519	2,435
1958	91,945	91,945	83,912	83,812	154,484	154,484	2,552
1959	92,125	91,213	82,699	81,077	150,484	147,533	

Table 4: Crippled Children's Services (Continued)

Year	Federal Grants[5]		Federal Expenditures[6]		Total Expenditures[8]		Number of Children[9]
	Current	Constant	Current	Constant	Current	Constant	
1960	92,794	90,091	96,036	93,239	156,266	151,715	2,553
1961	118,195	112,567	121,465	115,681	176,213	167,822	2,660
1962	125,967	118,837	125,957	118,827	170,992	161,313	2,675
1963	125,262	117,067	126,128	117,877	172,636	161,342	2,743
1964	147,086	134,941			197,823	181,489	2,902
1965	172,121	155,064			235,511	212,172	2,018
1966	163,199	143,157	158,357	138,910			2,982
1967	167,058	142,785			279,814	237,153	3,010
1968	187,337	153,555	185,694	152,208			3,329
1969	227,914	178,058			319,844	249,878	2,903
1970			185,694	126,080			2,803
1971							3,039
1972	203,254	139,215	170,208	126,080	450,559	308,602	3,226
1973	210,740	136,844	220,142	134,486			3,217
1974	221,900						

Appendix A: Sources for Primary Data on Vermont

[5]Data source 1937-1946 and 1968-1974 is the *Biennial Report of the Treasurer and Auditor of the State of Vermont*, respective years.   Data source 1947-1967 is compiled from *Annual Report of the United States Secretary of the Treasury*, respective years.

[6]Data source 1937-1955 is the *Biennial Report of the Treasurer and Auditor of the State of Vermont*, respective years.   Data source 1956-1972 is the *Biennial Report of the Vermont State Department of Health*, respective years.

[7]Data source for federal expenditures as above; state expenditure figures for all years derived from internal reports of the State Board of Health.   Financial statements for the divisions of Maternal and Child Health and of Public Health Nursing were combined until 1951 because "the public health nurses largely render the services which obtain the (MCH) results" (*11th Biennial Report of State Department of Public Health*).   The public health nurses also performed generalized nursing services in many towns, and some specialized in case-finding and follow-up for TB cases throughout the state.   The towns receiving generalized nursing services reimbursed the PHN division with small sums of money (*2nd Report of State Health Commission, 1951-52*), but the division's financing came predominantly from the US Public Health Services and from state MCH matching funds.

According to time-cost studies issued by the PHN division, it is "fair to assume" that since 1951 half of the PHN budget has financed MCH activities and about one-fifth of the total PHN budget has derived from federal MCH money.   Therefore, the total MCH expenditure figures are calculated as follows:

(1) 1937-1950 figures derived from adding state MCH expenditures to federal MCH expenditures.

(2) 1950-1965, 1967, 1969 and 1972 figures derived by adding total expenditure of MCH division (includes state and federal monies) to 1/2 of total expenditure for PHN division (includes state and federal MCH money).

Unfortunately, because MCH, CCS and Mental Health were
combined in 1963 into a new division called Child Health
Services, separate expenditure information on MCH and PHN
operations became only sporadically available.

[8]Data for 1937–1949 derived by adding federal CCS expenditures
(A and B funds) with state expenditures on Infantile Paralysis
as recorded in Audit Reports of the Vermont State Board of
Health (Health Department files), respective years. Data for
1950–1972 are compiled from internal expenditure reports of
the Vermont Board of Health, respective years.

[9]Data derived from figures compiled in periodic reports of the
Vermont Health Department to D/HEW in Washington, D.C.
(Foltz and Sacks, 1974).

Table 5:   Federal Grants to Connecticut's Title V Programs

	CCS		MCH	
Year	Current Dollars	Constant Dollars	Current Dollars	Constant Dollars
1936			31,034	72,679
1937			41,223	92,636
1938	33,735	76,845	37,281	84,923
1939	17,977	41,613	52,074	120,542
1940	31,671	72,144	65,322	148,797
1941	67,641	143,307	70,632	149,644
1942	75,453	142,364	55,320	104,377
1943	33,693	59,319	58,395	102,908
1944	72,458	124,498	57,539	98,964
1945	79,345	132,906	64,800	108,543
1946	68,206	102,258	80,860	121,229
1947	143,731	192,669	171,776	230,262
1948	86,245	108,348	85,585	107,591
1949	131,456	166,190	100,925	127,592
1950	134,837	168,126	97,434	121,489
1951	179,000	209,112	117,096	136,794
1952	177,200	202,514	119,064	136,073
1953	175,768	199,058	142,484	161,364
1954	182,906	204,136	124,300	138,728
1955	191,172	210,310	130,314	143,360
1956	211,683	225,195	144,763	154,003
1957	216,950	222,513	214,271	219,765
1958	214,457	214,457	257,922	257,922
1959	213,640	210,276	246,266	242,388
1960	221,340	214,269	259,346	251,061
1961	257,068	245,763	282,749	270,315
1962	286,180	270,491	356,556	337,073
1963	301,310	281,073	329,747	307,686
1964	203,024	277,596	382,737	351,619
1965	353,990	319,197	334,223	401,608
1966	384,907	337,934	573,117	502,999
1967	443,813	377,392	687,904	585,002
1968	447,555	365,948	720,902	589,454
1969	502,414	391,899	665,261	518,924
1970	512,098	378,770	690,127	510,298
1971	528,134	372,976	807,127	570,132
1972	531,100	363,518		

Table 6: Federal Grants to Vermont's Title V Programs

| | MCH | | CCS | |
Year	Current Dollars	Constant Dollars	Current Dollars	Constant Dollars
1937	23,313	52,984	12,217	27,766
1938	36,377	82,675	19,233	43,711
1939	38,981	90,653	18,410	42,814
1940	57,774	131,304	17,298	39,314
1941	60,115	127,904	23,070	43,528
1942	48,377	91,277	25,150	47,452
1943	61,649	108,156	20,917	36,789
1944	50,722	87,452	20,975	36,164
1945	51,812	86,353	15,916	26,527
1946			23,369	34,879
1947	74,450	99,267	35,214	46,952
1948	69,652	87,065	45,537	56,921
1949	53,811	68,115	52,417	66,351
1950	72,895	91,119	65,624	82,030
1951	80,601	93,722	77,205	89,773
1952	76,571	88,013	72,972	83,876
1953	87,615	99,562	100,028	113,668
1954	78,760	87,511	72,713	80,792
1955	71,102	78,134	64,037	70,370
1956	77,007	81,922	97,606	103,836
1957	100,313	103,415	97,263	100,271
1958	105,640	105,640	91,945	91,945
1959	107,217	105,115	92,125	91,213
1960	109,734	106,548	92,794	90,091
1961	120,184	114,461	118,195	112,567
1962	125,742	118,624	125,967	118,837
1963	128,721	120,300	125,262	117,067
1964	135,169	124,008	147,086	134,941
1965	137,635	123,995	172,121	155,064
1966	186,738	146,261	163,199	143,157
1967	177,114	150,097	167,058	142,785
1968	177,663	145,625	187,337	153,555
1969	177,585	138,738	227,914	178,058
1970	136,000	100,740		
1971	290,921	204,874		
1972	195,331	133,788	203,254	139,215
1973	205,772	133,618	210,740	136,844
1974	274,243		221,900	

Appendix B:

LOCATIONAL DATA

Appendix B: Locational Data

Table 1: Connecticut Towns Having MCH Well-Child Conferences*
(By absolute number of towns per county)

County	1940		1959		1971		(N Towns in County)	
	Urban	Rural	Urban	Rural	Urban	Rural	Urban	Rural
Fairfield	3	7	3	3	2	2	(8)	(15)
Hartford	6	12	1	7	1	7	(13)	(16)
Litchfield	0	19	0	4	0	7	(1)	(25)
Middlesex	0	12	3	6	0	3	(1)	(14)
New Haven	3	6	0	5	0	3	(14)	(13)
New London	1	10	0	11	0	13	(3)	(19)
Tolland	1	19	0	7	0	6	(1)	(12)
Windham	0	13	0	4	0	6	(0)	(15)
Total	14	88	7	47	3	47	(14)	(129)

*Connecticut data report the actual location of Well Child Conferences under the MCH program rather than the catchment areas of service recipients. Rural towns are those which in the 1960 Census had less than one inhabitant per acre; urban towns are those where population density equals or exceeds one inhabitant per acre.

Source: Tyler, 1973: 71-74.

Appendix B: Locational Data

Table 2: Vermont Towns Served by MCH Well-Child Conferences*
(By absolute number of towns per county)

County	1940		1960		1968		1974		(N Towns in County)	
	Urban	Rural	Urban	Rural	Urban	Rural	Urban	Rural	Urban	Rural
Addison	0	13	1	20	1	22	1	15	(1)	(24)
Bennington	0	2	0	10	0	13	0	14	(0)	(17)
Caledonia	0	4	0	14	0	17	0	16	(0)	(17)
Chittendon	0	7	0	15	1	14	1	7	(2)	(16)
Essex	0	4	0	13	0	14	0	9	(0)	(19)
Franklin	0	5	0	13	1	14	0	5	(1)	(16)
Grand Isle	0	3	0	5	0	5	0	0	(0)	(5)
La Moille	0	4	0	10	0	10	0	7	(0)	(10)
Orange	0	1	0	13	0	17	0	15	(0)	(17)
Orleans	0	0	1	11	1	16	1	16	(1)	(18)
Rutland	0	8	0	21	1	26	1	19	(1)	(27)
Washington	0	0	1	13	2	18	2	15	(2)	(19)
Windham	0	17	0	14	0	21	0	14	(0)	(23)
Winsor	0	7	0	17	0	24	0	13	(0)	(24)
Total	0	75	3	189	7	231	6	165	(8)	(252)

*Vermont data report the towns whose residents were actually treated at Well-Child Conferences although the WCCs themselves were not necessarily held in these towns. Unfortunately no information is available on actual location of the clinics. Again, by definition, rural towns are those which in the 1960 Census had less than one inhabitant per acre; urban towns are those where population density equals or exceeds one inhabitant per acre.

Source: *Biennial Reports of the Vermont State Department of Health* for 1940, 1960, and 1968; data for 1974 derived from internal activities records of the Vermont State Health Department in Burlington.

Appendix C

PROBLEMS OF DATA COLLECTION

A major challenge in using case studies is to
fit them into a theoretical framework. Case studies
are helpful for generating hypotheses that can be
systematically interrelated by theory. They are also
useful for illustrating and evaluating hypotheses.
But in order to generate hypotheses, or even to test
them, data must be obtained. These data may be
either qualitative or empirical, suggestive or
quantifiable. This appendix relates the methods by
which information on the state impacts of federal
health policy was obtained and utilized.

While billions of federal dollars have been
poured into the states to finance the general health
and welfare of the American people, little attention
has been paid to the coordinated effect of such
policy on the constituent states. Previous studies
have evaluated various discrete programs on an ad hoc
basis, but often they have neglected the contextual
environments and the overall intent of federal
policy. In our research, we utilized three broad
approaches to the analysis of policy: longitudinal,
synchronic, and comparative.

The first approach employed an historical
perspective on the development of health policy at
the federal level and within states. Therefore, we
relied on textual analyses of documents from primary
and secondary sources as the policy unfolded. The
second approach treated each state cross-sectionally
at different points in time. This approach entailed
a contextual analysis of the quantitative as well
as the qualitative data available. The third
approach compared two New England states (Connecticut
and Vermont) cross-sectionally and over time for
their similarities and contrasts. Throughout the
following descriptive review of our methodology we
address several basic questions. What types of data
were collected? How did we go about getting them?
Was access easy or difficult? How reliable were data
sources? And of what use were the data obtained?

At the national level, our data collection was
focused because we began with specific legislative
pronouncements about child care. With federal policy
as the point of departure, we sought evidence on its

94

specific intent and on how it was shaped within the
federal bureaucracy. Since we were not concerned
with federal policy-making per se but only with the
consequences of a specific policy, we sought limited
data from Congressional sources. The bulk of our
materials came from departmental sources.

On the legislative side, we looked at committee
reports, transcripts of hearings, conference
committee reports, and the legislative proposals
themselves. We also studied information on the
authorizing legislation for various child care
programs, the supplemental acts of Congress, and the
amounts of dollars in annual appropriations. In
addition, we relied on commentaries provided by the
Congressional Quarterly.

On the administrative side, we held interviews
with HEW officials and obtained their regulations,
guidelines, directives and letters of instruction.
We also obtained health surveys and health reports to
sketch the national scene of child care measures
throughout the United States, as well as in Connecticut and Vermont.

Since all the Congressional materials and the
federal regulations are published, such data were
easily available. Guidelines, letters of instruction, manuals and circulars were more difficult to
obtain, however, and there were surprising gaps in
the materials. For example, although Title XIX
(Medicaid) was added to the Social Security Act in
1965, no regulations were issued for several years
after the passage of the legislation. And no regulations were ever issued for the Maternity and Infant
Care Projects (1963), which have operated directly
from guidelines.

HEW officials in Washington and in the Boston
regional office readily shared their time, knowledge,
and materials with us. Such regional sources were
useful although we also found that duplicate
materials were available at D/HEW in Washington and
at the state health departments. Furthermore, the
Boston regional office, which basically receives and
transmits copies of documents, had only the most
recent letters on file.

We encountered greater problems when collecting
financial data and other quantitative indicators.

While information on authorizations and appropriations for any given program was readily available,
information actually proving disbursements of funds
was more difficult to obtain. Moreover, sources such
as the *Annual Reports of the U.S. Secretary of the
Treasury*, HEW's *Financial Assistance by Geographic
Area*, OEO's *Federal Outlays in Connecticut and
Vermont*, the *Social Security Bulletin*, and the
Statistical Abstract of the United States have
provided conflicting data on the amounts allocated
for the programs under study. Additional information
for Title V programs was also obtained from published
accounts of their early years and from HEW audits.

At the state level, financial information was
gathered from reports to the State Comptroller, and
from the Office of Federal-State Relations which
handled federal grants-in-aid. The Connecticut
Public Expenditure Council, through its periodic
publications, also provided valuable additional
information about Connecticut. In many instances,
however, these various accountings did not agree and,
despite many efforts, we found ourselves unable to
determine precisely how much federal money had been
spent in a specific program since its inception.

Information about state and local matching
funds proved equally elusive. State health agencies
need not provide a line-item accounting when
reporting to the federal government on Title V
formula grants. Fiscal data on earlier years were
easier to obtain because, until the mid-fifties,
financial data had been annually published in
detailed format in Connecticut's *Administrative
Report to the Governor* and its *Comptroller's Report*
and in Vermont's *Biennial Report of the Treasurer
and Auditor of the State of Vermont*. Thereafter,
publication of sucn materials ceased and only gross
information was recorded by the state reporting
systems. Segal and Fritschler's cautionary note is
most apt: "among the most unreliable statistics in
government today are those concerned with federal
grants-in-aid" (Segal and Fritschler, 1972).

Some of these difficulties in collecting
financial data are due to changes in the accounting
procedures, particularly after 1966. After that
year, line-item approval of budgetary items was no
longer required by HEW and some of the details

disappeared from the reports. During the years of line-item approval, budget revisions were commonplace and were designed, apparently, to sanction funds already expended. For example, in 1964 there were five revisions in Connecticut; in 1965, there were four. Also, special project budgets changed at least as often; in one year, there even were eight such revisions. Other indications of the "softness" of fiscal data are provided by several letters and memoranda attached to various documents, which suggest how easily funds were manipulated and shifted.

On a broader level, note should be taken of the changes in format for reporting policy results, and the problems these changes have entailed. If the format for reporting information had been changed, the question arose whether absolute changes really occurred in the pattern of services delivered or only in the way the facts were reported. Changes of format prohibit the collection of fully comparable material and, therefore, obscure the analysis of trends. This problem is common in other efforts to evaluate the quality of public services. It has applied to 'trends' in crime-rates for many years and the successes or failures they imply. But the problem is a bothersome one. Unfortunately, such changes in the format of state reporting have been due more to federal agency requirements than to state-level caprice. In this limited respect, there is a very clear federal impact on the state arena, but the outcome is more precedural than substantive.

Changes in the *quality* and *quantity* of health care are more appropriately reflected in aggregate data on medical and supportive services than in terms of financial largesse. But there was no indication of the quality of such services. An important initial aim of our study was to catalogue the demographic characteristics and health status of child populations in both states. From the decennial *Census*. we obtained information about whether children were poor or rich, urban or rural. From the *Registration Reports* and departmental reports to Washington, D.C., we mapped infant mortality rates by geographic area. The state health departments provided information on the location of hospitals, pediatric clinics, and visiting nurse associations. The Crippled Children and Medicaid programs supplied information on number of children

served. And from the AMA's computer tape of participating physicians, we learned about the geographic
distribution of pediatricians and other physicians
concerned with child health in Connecticut and
Vermont.

Questions still remain about which children got
which services, what was the unmet need, and how
prevalent were crippling diseases. These questions
cannot be answered inthe absence of refined,
systematic health surveys. Unfortunately, the data
available in national health surveys are valid only
for the whole country and not for any particular
constituent state. Such surveys assume a certain
average for the states and do not show variation of
state practices, nor do they show state or inter-
local variations.

In contrast to collecting information on policy
intentions at the federal level, the collection of
state-level data was much more complicated. We
sought information on reactions to federal intentions
and inputs, as well as on independent state policy
initiatives. Eventually our combined historical,
cross-sectional and comparative approaches produced
an inductive analysis of how Connecticut and Vermont
implemented several federal-state health programs.

We originally expected that federal health
policy would have provoked a variety of reactions
from state legislatures: anticipatory, responsive,
obstructive, supplementary, innovative. Therefore,
we examined the political histories of the General
Assemblies in Connecticut and Vermont since 1933 and
their performance over time. Statistics were
collected on the partisan composition of the legislative houses and on the political characteristics of
each state. We also gathered data on the total
numbers of bills annually proposed and annually
passed, with particular reference to health policy
issues. After examining all the bills proposed and
passed since 1933, and after classifying appropriate
items into one of twenty-one broadly defined health
and welfare categories,* we found that only a small

---

*These twenty-one categories were: (a) Intergovern-
mental Relations and Administrative Issues;
(b) Federal-State Relations; (c) Health Planning;
(d) Health Insurance; (e) Child Health; (f) Crippling
Diseases and Their Physical Treatment; (g) Maternal
Health; (h) Handicapped Children and Their Rehabili-

fraction of the annual proposals in either state
dealt with health policy issues.

From among the health-related bills, a number
were selected for follow-through by reading the
committee hearings. Although there were no obstacles
to access, obtaining these political data was a time-
consuming process. Published sources like the annual
Connecticut Register and Manual and the annual
Vermont Yearbook also provided background information
on the legislators who were frequent sponsors of
health legislation. These data on legislative
activities were suspect because the sources on
various years were occasionally inaccurate and incomplete. In addition, the Legislative Record Index,
the annual List of Bills, and the annual Printed
Bills tabulated different types of information.
Nonetheless, the materials available clearly
indicated a low salience for health policy issues
within the General Assembly of either state. And
these findings suggested that the influence and
impact of federal policy were to be found elsewhere.

Our study required a brief examination of each
state's political system as a whole in order to set
the legislative scene in perspective. The political
context was described by observing alternating
partisan control over the various state-wide elective
offices, the degree of competitiveness evident
during elections, and the organizational nature of
state political parties. Again, compilations of data
like the annual *Register and Manual*, the *Vermont
Yearbook* and the Council of States' *Book of the
States* were reliable and useful, as were secondary
analyses like Lockard's *New England State Politics*,
Fesler's *The Fifty States and Their Local Governments*,
and the Nuquists' *Vermont State Government and
Administration*.

---

*tation; (i) School Health; (j) Immunization;
(k) Public Health Nursing; (l) Child Welfare-ADC-
AFDC-Custodial Care; (m) Day Care; (n) Mental Retardation; (o) Nutrition; (p) Family Planning, Birth
Control and Abortion; (q) Child Abuse; (r) Fluorida-
tion; (s) Drugs and Liquor; (t) Prevention and
Safety; and (u) General Assistant and Public Welfare.

Each state has two agencies for implementing
federal and state child care policy: the health
department and the welfare department. As our study
progressed, the respective strengths and weaknesses,
as well as histories and futures, of these two
administrative departments became foci for enquiry
and comparison. The process by which public goals
and funds become transformed through these agencies
into health services is basically an administrative
one, and we sought to illuminate this process. Each
state library and the respective administrative
departments themselves provided most of the source
materials on administrative developments. We had
been warned by cooperative state officials not to
rely fully on their filing systems; all data sources
needed to be double-checked. Furthermore, we learned
that a state library, although the official deposi-
tory for state documents, does not always vigorously
pursue agencies to secure their delinquent reports.
Voluntary compliance with information-gathering
requirements and a cooperative spirit in record-
keeping are less evident at state levels, and these
short-comings have created serious deficiencies in
source materials.

The evidence that the respective departments
had undergone elaboration and change with the
passage of time was of particular importance. In
part, these transformations merely reflected natural
growth in an expanding society and economy, but they
were also partly due to federal inputs. The welfare
departments in particular parlayed their police role
in the care of delinquents into an active
intermediary role in the health-services delivery
system, especially through their statutory levels of
financial reimbursements and eligibility standards.

We studied reports on schemes for administrative
reorganization which preceded the New Deal and which
provided historical evidence of how and why federal
policies stimulated organizational change. Likewise,
we examined the periodic state publications which
detailed the yearly readjustments in state governments. Once again, as with the legal analysis of
legislation or the fiscal analysis of expenditures,
organizational analysis told only part of the story;
but it was a vital component of the overall picture
of how federal policy penetrates and restructures a
state government.

In addition to the written documents and published aggregate data, interpretive materials were gathered through discussions and interviews with officials at state headquarters and local service levels. The officials in Hartford, Montpelier, Burlington, and other parts of Connecticut and Vermont were generous with their time, cooperative and friendly, as had been their counterparts in Washington. We also probed a number of other, sundry sources for an added understanding of the health policy process in Connecticut and Vermont. These courses included local newspapers; state reporters; informational bulletins and pamphlets from health and welfare departments; and academic theses of students at Yale University and the University of Vermont.

The final major theme of our research was the influence of health lobbies on the initiation, implementation and evaluation of state health policies. For this theme, we studied a series of major, representative interest groups. These included professional associations of physicians and other health workers in each state; special-interest disease groups like the Cystic Fibrosis Association of Connecticut and the Vermont Association for the Crippled; and public interest research groups in Connecticut and Vermont. Information was obtained from their publications and from newspaper articles on their activities; and their leaders, both past and present, were interviewed. Obtaining descriptive data on all relevant groups was, of course, impossible, but our procedure allowed us to study a number of critical groups and to investigate several in depth.

SELECTED REFERENCES

Advisory Commission on Intergovernmental Relations
    1972-75   "Sub-state Regionalism and the Federal
            System," 5 Volumes, Washington, D.C.

    1974   "Federal-State-Local Finances: Significant
            Features of Fiscal Federalism,"
            Washington, D.C.

Alford, Robert R.
    1974   Health Care Politics: Ideological and
            Interest Group Barriers to Reform.
            Chicago: University of Chicago Press.

Altenstetter, Christa
    1971   "American Roulette" National Health Policy
            Making and Health Program Implementation."
            Working Paper No. 107-20, The Urban
            Institute, Washington, D.C.

    1973a   "A Brief Revised History of the Children's
            Bureau." Health Policy Project Working
            Paper No. 11, Yale University.

Altenstetter, Christa and James Warner Bjorkman
    1974   "The Impact of Federal Child Health
            Programs on State Health Policy Formation
            and Service Delivery: The Case of
            Connecticut." Presented at the Annual
            Meeting of the American Political Science
            Association, Chicago, 29 August -
            2 September.

    1976   "The Re-Discovery of Federalism: The
            Impact of Federal Child Health Programs on
            Connecticut State Health Policy Formation
            and Service Delivery" in Charles O. Jones
            and Robert Thomas, eds., Public Policy

103

Altenstetter and Bjorkman (Continued)
        Making in a Federal System, Beverly Hills,
        California, Sage Publications, Inc.:
        217-237.

American Medical Association
    1972   Distribution of Physicians, Hospitals and
            Hospital Beds in the U.S., Vol. I.

Averyt, William
    1973   "Connecticut Health Expenditures, 1961-
            1971," Health Policy Project Working Paper
            No. 10, Yale University.

Averyt, William, James Warner Bjorkman, and Anne-Marie
    Foltz
    1974   "Medical Professionals and Payment
            Policies: The Connecticut State Medical
            Society, 1930-1970." Health Policy Project
            Working Paper No. 18, Yale University.

Aycock, W.L.
    1924   "History of the Work of the Research
            Laboratory," Infantile Paralysis in
            Vermont: 1894-1922. Burlington: State
            Department of Public Health.

Bachrach, Peter and Morton S. Baratz
    1963   "Decisions and Non-decisions: An Analytic
            Framework." American Political Science
            Review, 57: 632-642.

Bailey, Stephen K.
    1950   Congress Makes a Law: The Story Behind the
            Unemployment Act of 1946. New York:
            Columbia University Press.

Bauer, Raymond and Kenneth Gergen, eds.
    1968   The Study of Policy Formation. New York:
            The Free Press.

Beer, Samuel H.
    1973   "The Modernization of American Federalism."
            Publius: The Journal of Federalism, 3:
            49-95.
Bjorkman, James Warner
    1973a   "Legislation and Sponsors in Connecticut:
            1930-1970." Health Policy Project Working
            Paper No. 7, Yale University.

Bjorkman, James Warner (Continued)
    1973b   "Government and Politics in Connecticut:
            1930-1970." Health Policy Project Working
            Paper No. 6, Yale University.

    1974   "Interest Groups in Connecticut's Health
            Policy Process: Some Preliminary
            Findings." Health Policy Project Working
            Paper No. 19, Yale University.

    1975a   "Interest Groups and Health Policy in
            Connecticut and Vermont: Who's Left in
            Charge of the Store?" Health Policy
            Project Working Paper No. 25, Yale
            University.

    1975b   "The Inconstant Design: Comparative Admin-
            istrative Histories of Health and Welfare
            Agencies in Two New England States." Health
            Policy Project Working Paper No. 17, Yale
            University.

Bjorkman, James Warner and Christa Altenstetter
    1973   "Descriptive Methodology: Scope, Themes,
            Approaches, Data Sources, Utility and
            Shortfalls." Health Policy Project Working
            Paper No. 14, Yale University.

Bjorkman, James Warner and Karen D. Kinsey
    1973   "The White House Conferences on Children
            and Youth: Seven Decades of Evolving
            National Policies." Health Policy Project
            Working Paper No. 1, Yale University.

Bradbury, Dorothy E.
    1962   Five Decades of Action for Children: A
            History of the Children's Bureau
            Washington, D.C.: U.S. D/HEW, Social
            Security Administration, Children's Bureau.

Brewer, Garry D. and James S. Kakalik
    1974   Improving Services to Handicapped Children:
            Summary and Recommendations. Prepared for
            D/HEW, Office of the Assistant Secretary
            for Planning and Evaluation, R-1402/1-HEW.
            Santa Monica, California: RAND (May).

Burns, Brian D.
    1972   "An Evaluation of the Reorganization of
            Vermont State Government, 1969-1972."
            (mimeographed).

Chen, Milton
    1975   "Federal Health Grants-in-aid to States:
            Rationale and Interstate Redistributional
            Impact." Health Policy Project Working
            Paper No. 28, Yale University.

Chen, Milton, James Bush, and Donald Patrick
    1975   "Social Indicators for Health Planning and
            Policy Analysis." Policy Sciences, 6, 1:
            71-89.

Citizen's Conference on State Legislatures
    1971   State Legislatures: An Evaluation of Their
            Effectiveness. New York: Praeger.

Cooper, Barbara S. and Nancy L. Worthington
    1975   "Comparison of Cost and Benefit Incidence
            of Government Medical Care Programs, Fiscal
            Years 1966 and 1969." U.S. D/HEW Publica-
            tion No. (SSA) 75-11852.

Dalston, Jeptha W.
    No   "Health Affairs and Politicians." Oklahoma
    Date   City: University of Oklahoma (mimeo-
            graphed).

Davis, Karen
    1975   "Medical Care for Mothers and Children--
            The Title V Programs." Washington, D.C.:
            The Brookings Institution (draft manu-
            script).

Derthick, Martha
    1968   "Inter-city Differences in Administration
            of the Public Assistance Program: The Case
            of Massachusetts," in James Q. Wilson, ed.,
            City Politics and Public Policy. New York:
            John Wiley and Louis, 243-266.

    1970   The Influence of Federal Grants: Public
            Assistance in Massachusetts. Cambridge:
            Harvard University Press.

106

Detore, John D.
    1965   "PHS Requirements Under the Civil Rights
            Act." Memorandum of the Executive Adminis-
            trator, Vermont State Department of Health
            (May 5).

Elazar, Daniel J.
    1972   American Federalism: A View From the
            States, Second Edition. New York: Thomas
            Crowell.

Eliot, Martha M.
    1972   "Six Decades of Action for Children."
            Children Today, 9: 2-6.

Fesler, James W.
    1967   The Fifty States and Their Local Govern-
            ments. New York: Alfred A. Knopf.

Foltz, Anne-Marie
    1974a   "The Impact of Federal Child Health Policy
            Under EPSDT: The Case of Connecticut,"
            Health Policy Project Report No. 3, Yale
            University.

    1975a   "The Development of Ambiguous Federal
            Policy: Early and Periodic Screening,
            Diagnosis and Treatment (EPSDT)." Health
            and Society: The Milbank Memorial Fund
            Quarterly, 53: 35-64.

Foltz, Anne-Marie and Donna Brown
    1975   "State Response to Federal Policy:
            Children, EPSDT and the Medicaid Muddle."
            Medical Care, 13: 630-642.

Foltz, Anne-Marie and Katie Sacks
    1974   "MCH Services Provided or Paid for by
            State or Local Official Public Health
            Agencies," compilations from reports filed
            with the Children's Bureau; Yale Health
            Policy Project files.

Friedman, Daniel H.
    1974   "Federal Policy Goals Under the Maternal
            and Child Health Legislation and the
            Responses of the State of Connecticut."
            Health Policy Project Working Paper No.
            21, Yale University.

Froman, Lewis A., Jr.
    1967   "An Analysis of Public Policies in Cities."
           Journal of Politics, 29: 94-108.

    1968   "The Categorization of Policy Contents,"
           in Austin Ranney, ed., Political Science
           and Public Policy: 41-52. Chicago:
           Markham Publishing Company.

George Washington University
    1973   Operational and Demographic Analysis for
           Maternal and Child Health Project.
           Washington, D.C.

Godfrey, E. Drexel, Jr.
    1949   The Transfer of the Children's Bureau.
           Washington, D.C.: Committee on Public
           Administration Cases.

Grad, F.O.
    1965   Public Health Law Manual. American Public
           Health Administration.

Grodzins, Morton
    1966   The American System. Edited by Daniel J.
           Elazar. Chicago: Rand McNally and
           Company.

Haveman, Robert H. and Robert D. Hamrin, editors
    1973   The Political Economy of Public Policy.
           New York: Harper & Row, Publishers.

Hinckley, Barbara
    1971   Stability and Change in Congress.
           New York: Harper and Row, Publishers.

Huron Institute
    1972   Federal Programs for Young Children: Review
           and Recommendations. Part I, Goals and
           Standards of Public Programs for Children.

Iglehart, John K.
    1974   "Health Report: HEW's Child Health
           Failure." National Journal Reports (June
           29): 969.

Janlon, J.L.
    1969   Principles of Public Health Administration,
           6th Edition. St. Louis: The C.V. Mosby
           Co.

Kakalik, James S., et al.
　　1973　Services for Handicapped Youth: A Program
　　　　　Overview. Prepared for D/HEW, Office of
　　　　　the Assistant Secretary for Planning and
　　　　　Evaluation, R-1220-HEW. Santa Monica,
　　　　　California: RAND (May).

　　1974　Improving Services to Handicapped Children.
　　　　　Prepared for D/HEW, Office of the Assistant
　　　　　Secretary for Planning and Evaluation, R-
　　　　　1420-HEW. Santa Monica, California: RAND
　　　　　(May).

Keniston, Kenneth
　　1974　"'Good Children' (Our Own), 'Bad Children'
　　　　　(Other People's), and the Horrible Work
　　　　　Ethic." Yale Alumni Magazine, XXXVII:
　　　　　6-10 (April).

Krizay, John and Andrew Wilson
　　1974　The Patient as Consumer. Lexington,
　　　　　Massachusetts: Lexington Books.

Lasswell, Harold D. and Abraham Kaplan
　　1950　Power and Society: A Framework for Politi-
　　　　　cal Inquiry. New Haven: Yale University
　　　　　Press.

Leach, Richard
　　1973　"Federalism: A Battery of Questions."
　　　　　Publius: The Journal of Federalism,
　　　　　3: 11-47.

Levenson, Rosalyn
　　1966　County Government in Connecticut: Its
　　　　　History and Demise. Stors, Connecticut:
　　　　　Institute of Public Service.

Lockard, Duane
　　1966　New England State Politics. Princeton,
　　　　　N.J.: Princeton University Press.

Lowi, Theodore J.
　　1964　"American Business, Public Policy, Case
　　　　　Studies and Political Theory." World
　　　　　Politics, XV: 677-715.

　　1972　"Four Systems of Policy, Politics, and
　　　　　Choice." Public Administration Review,
　　　　　XXXII: 298-310.

Lowi, Theodore J. (Continued)
  1973   "What Political Scientists Don't Need to
          Ask About Policy Analysis." Policy Studies
          Journal, 2: 61-67.

Mayhew, David R.
  1974   Congress: The Electoral Connection.   New
          Haven: Yale University Press.

Minnesota Systems Research
  No   "Health Care to Children: Current Programs
  Date   and Proposed Legislation." Project Report
          Series, No. 2-3 (7), mimeographed.

Morehouse, Thomas A.
  1972   "The Problem of Measuring the Impacts of
          Social Action Programs." Institute of
          Social, Economic, and Government Research,
          Occasional Paper No. 6. Fairbanks, Alaska:
          University of Alaska.

Murphy, Jerome T.
  1973   "Grease the Squeaky Wheel: A Report of the
          Implementation of Title V of the Elementary
          and Secondary Education Act of 1965, Grants
          to Strengthen State Departments of
          Education." Harvard Graduate School of
          Education, mimeographed. Cambridge,
          Massachusetts.

Novak, Barbara J.
  1973   "The Cystic Fibrosis Association of
          Connecticut, Inc. -- Notes on a Special
          Interest Group in Action." Health Policy
          Project Working Paper No. 12, Yale
          University.

Nuquist, Andrew and R. Nuquist
  1966   Vermont State Government and Administra-
          tion: A History and Descriptive Study of
          the Living Past. Burlington, Vermont:
          Government Research Center, University of
          Vermont.

Oettinger, Katherine B.
  1962   "A Half Century of Progress for All
          Children." The Child. 9: 43-51.

Ogle, David B.
1970   Strengthening the Connecticut Legislature.
         New Brunswick, N.J.:   Rutgers University
         Press.

Ostrom, Vincent
1973   "Can Federalism Make a Difference?"
         Publius: The Journal of Federalism,
         3: 197-237.

Peterson, Eric
1975   "Legal Challenges to Bureaucratic Discre-
         tion: The Influence of Lawsuits on the
         Implementation of EPSDT." Health Policy
         Project Working Paper No. 27, Yale
         University.

Pressman, Jeffrey L. and Aaron Wildavsky
1972   Implementation. Berkeley: University of
         California Press.

Redman, Eric
1973   The Dance of Legislation. New York:
         Simon and Schuster.

Russell, Viola
1957   A Chronological History of the Vermont
         Department of Health. Burlington, Vermont.

Schaefer, Guenther F. and Stuart H. Rakoff
1970   "Politics, Policy and Political Science:
         Theoretical Alternatives." Politics and
         Society, I: 51-77.

Schmidt, William M.
1973   "The Development of Health Services for
         Mothers and Children in the United States."
         American Journal of Public Health, 63: 425.

Segal, Morley and A. Lee Fritschler
1972   "Intergovernmental Relations and Contempor-
         ary Political Science: Developing an Inte-
         grative Typology." Publius: The Journal
         of Federalism, II: 95-122.

Sharkansky, Ira
1970   Regionalism and American Politics.
         Indianapolis and New York: Bobbs-Merrill
         Company, Inc.

Sharkansky, Ira (Continued)
1972   The Maligned States: Policy Accomplish-
        ments, Problems, and Opportunities.
        New York: McGraw-Hill Book Company.

1975   The United States: A Study of a Developing
        Country. New York: David McKay Company,
        Inc.

Shaw, Gaylord
1973   "Government as Promoter, Sustainer, and
        Subsidizer and Private Enterprise." in
        Haveman and Hamrin, op. cit.: 47-51.

Silver, George A.
1974   "Impact of Federal Child Health Legislation
        in the State of Connecticut." Health
        Policy Project Report No. 1, Yale
        University.

1975   "The Hands of Esau: Reflections on
        Federalism and Child Health Services in the
        United States" (Sun Valley Forum).

Steiner, Gilbert
1976   The Children's Cause. Washington, D.C.:
        Brookings Institute

Stevens, Robert and Rosemary Stevens
1974   Welfare Medicine in America: A Case Study
        of Medicaid. New York: The Free Press.

Stevens, Rosemary
1971   American Medicine and the Public Interest.
        New Haven: Yale University Press.

Stevens, Rosemary and Robert Stevens
1970   "Medicaid: Anatomy of a Dilemma." Law and
        Contemporary Problems: 348-425.

Stoga, Alan
1975   "Fiscal Federalism in Connecticut: The
        Economic Impact of Grants-in-Aid." Health
        Policy Project Working Paper No. 26, Yale
        University.

Tyler, Natalie C.
1973   "The Well-Child Conference: A Reflection
        of the Nation's Policy Toward Children at
        the National and State Level." Health

Tyler, Natalie C. (Continued)
        Policy Project Working Paper No. 15, Yale
        University.

U.S. Civil Service Commission
    1963   "State Salary Survey, July 1." Washington,
            D.C.

    1973   "State Salary Survey, July 1." Washington,
            D.C.

Vineyard, Dale
    1976   "Rediscovery of the Aged: 'Senior Power'
            and Public Policy." Paper presented at the
            Annual Meeting of the American Political
            Science Association, Chicago, 2-5 Septembe
            September.

Walker, David
    1974   "How Fares Federalism in the Mid-
            Seventies?" Annals of the American Academy
            of Political and Social Science,
            416 (November): 17-31.

Wallace, Helen M.
    1962   Health Services for Mothers and Children.
            Philadelphia: W.B. Sanders Company.

Wholey, Joseph S.
    1969   The Absence of Program Evaluation as an
            Obstacle to Effective Public Expenditure
            Policy: A Case Study of Child Health Care
            Programs. Washington, D.C.: The Urban
            Institute.

Wholey, Joseph S. and George A. Silver
    1966   "Maternal and Child Health Care Programs."
            Washington, D.C.: HEW, Office of the
            Assistant Secretary for Program Coordina-
            tion.

Witte, E.E.
    1963   The Development of the Social Security Act.
            Madison: University of Wisconsin Press.

Wright, Deil
    1974   "Intergovernmental Relations: An
            Analytical Overview." The Annals of the
            American Academy of Political and Social
            Science, (November): 1-16.

ABOUT THE AUTHORS

Christa Altenstetter, Research Fellow at the International Institute of Management in Berlin and Associate Professor of Political Science at the City University of New York, received her political science doctorate in 1967 at Heidelberg University where she taught political science from 1967 to 1968. She has

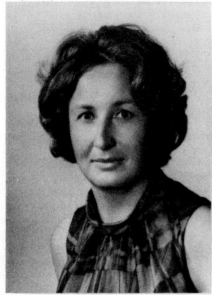

also taught and/or researched at Harvard University, the Urban Institute in Washington, D.C., Syracuse University, Yale University, Kiel University, the Fogarty International Center at the National Institutes of Health, and American University. Author of *Der Föderalismus in Österreich,* 1945-1968, "Planning for Health Facilities in the United States and West Germany," *Organizations for Managing National Hospital Planning Programs: A Comparison of France and the Federal Republic of Germany;* "Medical Interests and the Public Interest: A German-American Comparison," *Health Policy Making and Administration in West Germany and the United States,* "Intergovernmental Profiles in Austria and West Germany: A Comparative Perspective," *Health Planning Methods for Ambulatory Care: The Case of the Federal Republic of Germany;* and "Wohnunterkünfte, Arbeitsplätze und Schulen für ethnische Minderheiten in Ballungsräumen: Ein Deutsch-Amerikanischer Vergleich," her current research interests encompass the politics and organization of health planning processes in comparative perspective.

James Warner Bjorkman, Assistant Professor of Political Science and Preventive Medicine at the University of Wisconsin--Madison, received his Ph.D. in Political Science from Yale University in 1976. Currently associated with the Program in Health Services Administration, he was Research Associate at

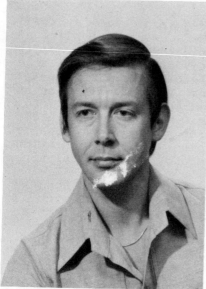

the Indian Institute of Public Administration (New Delhi) during 1970-1972 and Research Staff Scientist on the Health Policy Project in the Yale School of Medicine's Department of Epidemiology and Public Health during 1973-1976. He has authored several articles on Indian public policies as well as *The Politics of Administrative Alienation: Relations Among Civil Servants and Political Leaders in India's Rural Development Programs;* and, with Christa Altenstetter, he has published "The Rediscovery of Federalism: The Impact of Federal Programs on Connecticut's State Health Policy Formation and Service Delivery;" "Accountability in Health Care: An Essay on Mechanisms, Muddles, and Mires;" and "Policy, Politics and Child Health: Four Decades of Federal Initiative and State Response." His current research focuses on comparative public policies for representation and decentralization in British, Swedish and American health affairs as well as on comparative public policies for delivering rural health care in Third World countries.

116